DASH DIET COOKBOOK FOR BEGINNERS 2024

Unlock the Secrets to Lower Blood Pressure and Embrace Vibrant Health with Quick Tasty Recipes for Your Busy Life. Maximize Wellness and Minimize Kitchen Hours

Stefy Dennis

Table of Contents

Bonus

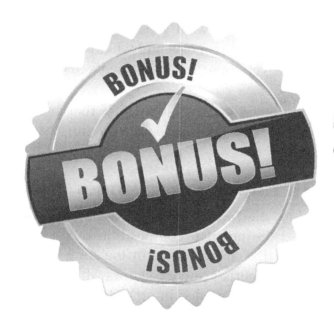

Let's start the Dash Diet!

Scan the QR Code and enjoy your free bonus!

GET YOUR FREE GIFT

Introduction

The DASH diet offers a refreshing approach to achieving your health goals. It stands out by promoting sustainable and straightforward eating habits, rooted in scientific research, that empower you to reach your objectives without sacrificing the enjoyment of delicious food. Unlike restrictive fad diets that often promise rapid results but struggle to deliver in the long term, the DASH diet prioritizes gradual yet effective changes to your existing dietary habits.

Rather than imposing stringent rules and forcing you to bid farewell to your favorite foods, the DASH diet encourages you to form simple adjustments that align with your physical well-being. It doesn't dictate a one-size-fits-all approach but instead empowers you to find what works best for you within its guidelines. This flexibility makes it easy to incorporate DASH principles into your daily life.

When you embark on your DASH journey, you'll discover that there's no singular "right" way to follow the diet. Instead, you'll have the freedom to tailor it to your preferences and unique needs. As you become more mindful of the choices you make regarding what goes into your body, you'll gain a deeper understanding of what should be included in your meals and what can be omitted. This heightened awareness empowers you to form subtle yet impactful adjustments to counter any unhealthy tendencies you may have developed.

In essence, the DASH diet is not a temporary solution but a sustainable lifestyle that encourages you to form choices that support your overall well-being. It's a path to healthier eating that allows you to relish the journey and savor the flavors along the way.

What is the DASH diet and why is it important to understand?

The DASH (Dietary Approaches to Stop Hypertension) diet, which is supported by the National Heart, Lung, and Blood Institute in the US, analyzes the nutrient composition of various food products in order to develop specific dietary patterns that are effective in lowering high blood pressure. The diet is the product of the ingenuity of bio scientists and legislators who collaborated to identify the components of a person's diet that need to be excluded in order to bring the rate of rise in blood pressure under control.

The amount of people who have complained of having high blood pressure has nearly doubled in the past two decades, which is what led to the development of the DASH diet. As a result of this, medical professionals, in collaboration with the US Department of Health and Human Services, have been researching hypertension and the many hazards that are connected with having high blood pressure in an effort to identify effective treatments for the condition. After conducting an in-depth investigation, the researchers came to the conclusion that those who pursued a plant-based diet or who preferred to consume a greater quantity of vegetables exhibited less indicators and instances of their blood pressure increasing. The DASH diet was developed with this understanding as its primary principle.

A person who follows the DASH diet prioritizes eating foods that are minimally processed and have a higher organic content. This method of dieting emphasizes the consumption of lean meats, whole grains, fruits, and vegetables as its primary food groups. In extreme circumstances, the individual showing major indicators of heart-related ailments due to high blood pressure is also encouraged to become vegan for a while to lessen concerns associated to hypertension. This is being done in an attempt to reduce the likelihood of problems related to hypertension.

In addition to this, the diet prescribes a very particular way to consume salt. The dietary rules of the DASH diet greatly minimize the amount of salt that is consumed. This is done since excessive amounts of salt and oil both greatly increase the blood pressure that is found in the human body. The dishes that are recommended for consumption on the DASH diet are composed of healthy ingredients including leafy green vegetables, natural fruits, low-fat dairy products, and lean proteins like chicken, fish, and a great deal of beans. In addition to reducing the amount of salt that is consumed, the general rule of thumb is to consume less food that is high in processed carbohydrates, red meat, and composite fat. If you adhere to the DASH diet, it is recommended that you do not consume in excess of one tsp (2,300 mg) of sodium in a single day. This recommendation is in accordance with conventional practice.

The diet is not only recommended by the US Department of Agriculture (USDA), but it is also completely risk-free to follow. The DASH diet was added in the United States Dietary Guidelines as one of the three healthy diets that are recommended from 2015-2020.

The Science Behind DASH: How It Benefits Your Health

To comprehend the significance of the DASH diet, it's essential to grasp the scientific foundations that make it a valuable tool for improving health. The DASH diet was originally developed by the National Heart, Lung, and Blood Institute (NHLBI) in the United States as a response to the growing concern over hypertension, a major risk factor for heart disease and stroke. It was designed to be a dietary strategy that would effectively lower blood pressure, but as subsequent research has shown, its benefits extend far beyond blood pressure management.

The DASH diet's fundamental ideas, which place an emphasis on eating foods high in nutrients while consuming little sodium, are at its foundation. It promotes eating a diet rich in fruits, vegetables, whole grains, dairy products, and lean proteins on a regular basis. These foods are naturally low in saturated fats and cholesterol and provide essential nutrients like potassium, calcium, magnesium, and fiber. The diet also encourages reducing the consumption of high-sodium foods, particularly processed and fast foods, which are notorious for contributing to hypertension.

One of the key reasons why the DASH diet matters is its remarkable ability to lower blood pressure. Strong scientific evidence backs up this assertion. Numerous studies, including the original DASH trial conducted in the 1990s, have consistently demonstrated that individuals who adhere to the DASH diet experience significant reductions in their blood pressure levels. This reduction in blood pressure is attributed to several factors, including the higher intake of potassium, which counteracts the effects of sodium on blood pressure, and the overall improvement in the quality of one's diet.

However, the benefits of the DASH diet extend beyond blood pressure management. This has been linked to a decreased risk of cardiovascular disease, which stands as the primary cause of death globally. The emphasis on whole, nutrient-dense foods in the DASH diet promotes heart health by lowering LDL (bad) cholesterol levels and improving overall lipid profiles. Consequently, this lowers the likelihood of developing atherosclerosis and coronary artery disease.

Moreover, the DASH diet aligns with principles that can aid in weight management and diabetes prevention. Its emphasis on portion control and the consumption of foods that are filling yet lower in calories makes it a sensible choice for individuals looking to maintain a healthy weight or shed excess pounds. Furthermore, the diet's focus on whole grains and foods with a low glycemic index aids with blood sugar regulation, which is essential for both managing and preventing diabetes.

Another compelling aspect of the DASH diet is its role in promoting long-term dietary sustainability and overall well-being. Unlike many restrictive diets that are difficult to maintain over time, the DASH diet offers a balanced and realistic approach to eating. It encourages the enjoyment of a wide variety of foods, including those rich in flavor and nutrients, which can enhance adherence and satisfaction.

Moreover, the DASH diet is a lifetime commitment to better eating practices rather than just a temporary solution. Its focus on educating individuals about making better food choices fosters a deeper understanding of nutrition and empowers them to take control of their health. By instilling these principles, the DASH diet equips people with the tools they need to form informed dietary decisions that benefit them in the long run.

In an era where chronic diseases like hypertension, heart disease, and diabetes are on the rise, the DASH diet offers a practical and evidence-based solution. It serves as a beacon of hope for those seeking to take charge of their health through diet and lifestyle changes. Its emphasis on whole, natural foods and the reduction of processed and sodium-laden options aligns with the broader movement towards cleaner, healthier eating patterns.

The DASH diet is not just another dietary trend but a scientifically validated approach to improving health. Given its potential to lower blood pressure, lessen the risk of cardiovascular disease, help with weight management, and enhance general well-being, it is a dietary approach that people of all ages should think about. The DASH diet reminds us that the path to better health begins with the food we put on our plates and the choices we make every day. In a world where health challenges abound, the DASH diet stands as a beacon of hope, offering a practical and sustainable way to enhance our quality of life through better nutrition.

Assessing Your Health

In our journey towards better health, the first and most crucial step is to assess our current state of well-being. This process of self-evaluation serves as the foundation upon which we can build healthier and more fulfilling lives. By gaining a comprehensive understanding of our health, we can identify areas that require improvement, set achievable goals, and embark on a path towards positive change. Here, we will explore the key components of health assessment, including the measurement of blood pressure, considerations related to weight, cholesterol levels, and more.

Knowing Your Blood Pressure: The First Step

One of the foundational aspects of health assessment involves gaining insight into your blood pressure. Blood pressure, often known as BP, is a measurement of the force your blood exerts on your artery walls while it flows throughout your body. This measure is typically denoted as two numbers: systolic pressure (the higher of the two) and diastolic pressure (the lower of the two), with units expressed in millimeters of mercury (mm Hg).

Systolic pressure characterizes the force generated when your heart contracts and pumps blood into your arteries, while diastolic pressure signifies the pressure when your heart is in a resting state between beats. Generally, a standard blood pressure reading is recognized as approximately 120/80 mm Hg, though slight variations may occur based on individual factors.

It's critical to understand your blood pressure because high blood pressure, or hypertension, is sometimes referred to as the "silent assassin." This nickname originates from its capacity to develop quietly, without apparent symptoms, yet it can result in significant health complications like heart disease, stroke, and kidney problems if not managed effectively. Regular blood pressure monitoring is indispensable for early detection and timely intervention, as hypertension can be controlled through lifestyle modifications, medications, or a combination of both.

To gauge your blood pressure, you have the option of using a home blood pressure monitor or seeking assistance from a healthcare professional. It is advisable to measure your blood pressure at various times and under different circumstances to obtain a more precise assessment of your cardiovascular health. If your blood pressure consistently registers above the normal range, it is imperative to consult with a healthcare provider to devise a comprehensive management and reduction plan.

Other Health Considerations: Weight, Cholesterol, and More

In addition to monitoring your blood pressure, there are several other critical health considerations that play a pivotal role in assessing your overall well-being.

Weight: Keeping a healthy weight is crucial for lowering the risk of chronic illnesses including diabetes, heart disease, and some types of cancer. Body weight is a major predictor of health. The Body Mass Index (BMI) is a common tool used to assess weight relative to height, but it has limitations as it does not account for factors like muscle mass and body composition. Still, it can give you a general idea of whether you are obese, overweight, average weight, or underweight. It is important to remember that individual health varies, and discussions with a healthcare provider about your weight and its implications for your health are valuable.

Cholesterol Levels: Cholesterol is a waxy substance found in the cells of your body and in the foods you eat. Although LDL (low-density lipoprotein) cholesterol is essential for various bodily functions, an excess of it, often dubbed "bad" cholesterol, can accumulate in your arteries and contribute to the progression of atherosclerosis, which encompasses the narrowing and hardening of the arteries. This may make heart disease and stroke more likely. Conversely, HDL (high-density lipoprotein) cholesterol, which is sometimes referred to as "good" cholesterol, aids in the removal of LDL cholesterol from the bloodstream. Regular cholesterol checks can provide insights into your heart health and guide dietary and lifestyle choices.

Blood Sugar: Consistently checking your blood sugar levels is essential to assess your vulnerability to diabetes, a chronic condition distinguished by elevated blood sugar levels. Elevated blood sugar levels can give rise to complications like nerve damage, kidney issues, and vision impairment. Two frequently employed tests for measuring blood sugar levels and diagnosing diabetes or prediab.

Family Medical History: Your family's medical history can be a valuable resource for understanding your own health risks. Some people are more susceptible to certain diseases, such diabetes, cancer, or heart disease, due to certain genetic variables. A thorough discussion with family members about their health histories can provide insights and guide preventive measures.

Overall Lifestyle: Assessing your health goes beyond numerical values and medical tests. It also entails assessing the lifestyle decisions you make about nutrition, exercise, sleep patterns, stress reduction, and drug usage. These lifestyle factors have a profound impact on your health and well-being and are often within your control to modify for the better.

The Importance of Setting Clear Health Goals

Once you have gathered information about your health status, the next crucial step is setting clear health goals. These goals present as a roadmap for making positive changes and improvements in your well-being. Setting health goals is a powerful tool for motivation and accountability.

Well-defined health objectives ought to be time-bound, relevant, measurable, achievable, and specific (SMART). For example, instead of stating a general objective like "I want to lose weight," a SMART goal would be something like "I aim to lose 10 pounds in the next three months by increasing my daily physical activity to almost 30 minutes and reducing my daily calorie intake."

Here are some key reasons why setting clear health goals is important:

1. **Direction:** Health goals provide a clear sense of direction and purpose. They assist you in setting priorities related to your health and well-being.

2. **Motivation:** Goals present as a source of motivation and inspiration. When you have a specific target to work toward, you are more likely to stay committed to making positive changes in your life.

3. **Accountability:** Goals create accountability. When you set goals, you are more inclined to track your progress and hold yourself responsible for your actions and choices.

4. **Measurement:** Clear goals are measurable, allowing you to track your progress objectively. This measurement enables you to celebrate your successes and make adjustments when necessary.

5. **Adaptability:** Goals can be adjusted as needed. If you find that a goal is too challenging or not challenging enough, you can modify it to better align with your capabilities and aspirations.

6. **Empowerment:** Setting and achieving health goals can empower you to take control of your health and make informed choices that enhance your overall quality of life.

Evaluating your health is an essential first step in achieving better wellbeing. Understanding factors like blood pressure, weight, cholesterol levels, and blood sugar provides a comprehensive view of your health status. Additionally, recognizing the significance of family medical history and lifestyle choices adds depth to your assessment. Equipped with this knowledge, setting clear and SMART health goals empowers you to take deliberate actions toward a healthier, happier life. Remember that your health is a lifelong journey, and each step you take towards better health is a step in the right direction.

The DASH Diet Basics

The DASH diet is a powerful and evidence-based dietary strategy designed to promote better health, particularly in the context of managing blood pressure and reducing the risk of heart disease. In this chapter, we will delve into the fundamental principles of the DASH diet, offering insight into the various food groups it emphasizes, the importance of portion control, and how to navigate nutrition labels effectively. Understanding these vital aspects will empower you to fully utilize the potential of the DASH diet in enhancing your well-being.

The DASH Diet Food Groups: What to Eat and What to Limit

Allowed and Recommended Foods on the DASH Diet:

1. **Fruits:** Incorporate a variety of fruits, such as berries, apples, oranges, and bananas. These provide essential vitamins, minerals, and fiber.
2. **Vegetables:** Consume a wide range of colorful vegetables, including leafy greens, carrots, broccoli, and bell peppers. They contain abundant vitamins, minerals, and fiber.
3. **Whole Grains:** Opt for whole grains like brown rice, whole wheat bread, oats, and quinoa. These are high in fiber and nutrients.
4. **Lean Proteins:** Include sources of lean protein like skinless poultry, fish, lean cuts of beef or pork, and plant-based options like beans, lentils, and tofu.
5. **Dairy:** Opt for dairy products with reduced or no fat content, including yogurt, milk, and cheese. These selections are rich sources of calcium and protein.
6. **Nuts, Seeds, and Legumes:** Enjoy small portions of unsalted nuts & seeds, such as almonds, walnuts, and flaxseeds. Beans and lentils, both legumes, also make superb options.
7. **Fats:** Use healthy fats in moderation, such as olive oil, canola oil, and avocado. These provide heart-healthy monounsaturated fats.
8. **Fish:** Rich in omega-3 fatty acids, fatty fish such as trout, salmon, and mackerel promote heart health. Aim to consume these almost twice a week.
9. **Herbs & Spices:** Use spices and herbs to flavor your food instead of salt. This lowers salt intake.

Unallowable Foods on the DASH Diet:

To maximize the benefits of the DASH diet, it's crucial to avoid certain foods that can negatively impact your health:

1. **Fast Food:** Fast food usually contains excessive unhealthy fats, sodium, and empty calories, which do not align with the objectives of the DASH diet.
2. **High-Fat, Industrial Seed Oils:** These oils are frequently present in processed and fried foods and can contribute to inflammation and heart disease. It is crucial to steer clear of them for the sake of heart health.

3. **Lard:** Lard is a saturated fat source that should be eliminated from your diet to maintain low saturated fat intake.

4. **Prepackaged Foods High in Sugar/Sodium/Chemicals:** Processed foods often contain excessive sugar, sodium, and harmful chemicals. Avoid these products to keep your diet wholesome and heart-healthy.

5. **Red Meat in Excess of 2 Six-Ounce Portions a Week:** While red meat can be included in moderation, consuming it beyond 2 six-oz. servings a week may lead to a higher consumption of saturated fat, which is bad for the heart.

6. **Table Sugar:** Reduce your consumption of table sugar, as excessive sugar intake can contribute to health problems such as obesity and high blood pressure.

7. **Sodium in Excess of 2,300 mg a Day:** To sustain healthy blood pressure levels, restrict your daily sodium intake to 2,300 mg or less. The DASH diet aims to treat hypertension, a disorder that is linked to high sodium intake.

Portion Control: Managing Serving Sizes Effectively

Beyond prioritizing the right food groups, the DASH diet places significant importance on controlling portion sizes. If overindulged in, even healthful foods can cause weight gain and other health problems. It is essential to comprehend portion sizes in order to reach and stay at a healthy weight.

To assist people in making well-informed decisions about how much to consume, the DASH diet offers guidelines for portion control. These guidelines are typically based on daily calorie intake and can be customized to individual needs. For example, a typical DASH diet may recommend:

- **Grains:** 6-8 servings per day (based on a 2,000-calorie diet). A serving is roughly equivalent to one slice of bread or 1/2 teacup of cooked rice or pasta.
- **Vegetables:** 4-5 servings per day. A serving is about 1 teacup of raw leafy greens or 1/2 teacup of cooked vegetables.
- **Fruits:** 4-5 servings per day. A serving is typically 1 medium-sized fruit or 1/2 teacup of canned or severed fruit.
- **Dairy:** 2-3 servings per day. A serving might consist of 1 teacup of milk or yogurt.
- **Proteins:** two or fewer portions of fish, poultry, or lean meats each day. A serving weighs around three ounces, or about the same as a deck of cards.
- **Nuts, Seeds, and Legumes:** 4-5 portions each week. A serving may be equivalent to 1/3 teacup of nuts or 1/2 teacup of cooked legumes.
- **Fats and Oils:** 2-3 servings per day. A serving could be 1 tsp of oil or 1 tbsp of salad dressing.
- **Sweets:** Limited to 5 or fewer servings per week.

You may more effectively regulate your calorie intake and make sure you're getting the proper ratio of nutrients by being aware of these portion management guidelines.

Reading Labels: Navigating Nutrition Information

In today's food landscape, many packaged and processed foods line the supermarket shelves, making it essential to become a savvy label reader. The DASH diet promotes the practice of carefully examining nutrition labels to form informed decisions about the foods you buy and consume.

When reading labels, pay attention to the following key elements:

1. **Serving Size:** The serving size indicated on the label holds great importance, as all the nutritional details provided are contingent on this serving size. Exercise caution regarding portion sizes to prevent excessive consumption.

2. **Calories:** The calorie content per serving is indicated on the label. This information helps you gauge the energy value of the food.

3. **Nutrients:** Check the label for nutrients like total fat, cholesterol, saturated fat, trans fat, dietary fiber, sodium, carbohydrates, sugars, and protein. Limit your intake of trans fat, cholesterol, saturated fat, and sodium while upping your consumption of dietary fiber.

4. **Percent Daily Value (%DV):** The percentage of a nutrient that a serving of food contains provides to a daily diet based on a conventional 2,000-calorie diet is indicated by the %DV on the label. This can be a helpful reference point for assessing the nutritional significance of the food.

5. **Ingredients:** Examine the ingredient list to identify any added sugars or unhealthy fats, such as hydrogenated oils. Ingredients are typically arranged in descending order of quantity, so exercise caution if you find unhealthy components near the top of the list.

6. **Nutrition Claims:** Pay attention to nutrition claims on the packaging, such as "low in sodium" or "high in fiber." These claims can provide valuable information about the product's nutritional profile.

7. **Sodium Content:** Given the DASH diet's emphasis on reducing sodium intake, be particularly vigilant about the sodium content in packaged foods. Choose low-sodium or no-salt-added options when available.

Incorporating label reading into your shopping routine can help you make healthier choices and stay aligned with the DASH diet's principles.

Getting Started with DASH

In this chapter, we'll guide you through the initial steps of adopting the DASH Diet, helping you create an action plan, stock your DASH-friendly kitchen, and make meal planning a breeze.

Creating Your DASH Diet Action Plan

Creating your DASH Diet action plan is a critical first step toward adopting a heart-healthy lifestyle. It involves setting clear goals, seeking professional guidance, assessing your current diet, and making gradual changes. Let's explore each of these steps in more detail to help you get started on your DASH journey:

Set Clear Goals

- Begin by defining your health objectives. Whether you're looking to lower your blood pressure, improve heart health, or manage your weight, having clear goals will guide your DASH plan.
- Specific goals, such as reducing sodium intake or incorporating more vegetables into your diet, will give you a roadmap for making meaningful changes.

Consult a Healthcare Professional

- Before embarking on significant dietary changes, it's wise to consult a healthcare provider or registered dietitian. They are qualified to offer tailored advice depending on your particular medical requirements.
- A healthcare professional can assess your current health status, offer guidance on managing chronic conditions, and help you tailor the DASH Diet to your specific requirements.

Assess Your Current Diet

Take a close look at your current eating habits to gain insight into areas where improvements are needed. Consider the following aspects:

- Sodium Intake: Assess how much salt you consume daily and identify sources of high sodium in your diet. Reducing sodium is a core component of the DASH Diet.
- Fruit and Vegetable Consumption: Evaluate your intake of fruits and vegetables. Aim to increase these nutrient-rich foods in your meals and snacks.
- Protein Sources: Examine your sources of protein. Seek for chances to select lean foods such as tofu, skinless chicken, fish, and lentils.
- Sugar and Processed Foods: Identify sources of added sugars and processed foods in your diet, and work on reducing their consumption.

Gradual Transition

- Transitioning to the DASH Diet doesn't have to be an abrupt change. It's more sustainable to set achievable milestones and gradually incorporate DASH principles into your daily routine.
- Make modest, doable adjustments to your meals and snacks to start, then progressively build on your accomplishments over time.

Keep a Food Journal:

- For a few days, keeping a food journal can reveal important information about your eating habits. Keep track of everything you consume, including the serving sizes.
- Review your food diary to identify areas where you can make healthier choices and reduce less nutritious options.

Stay Accountable:

- Sharing your DASH goals with a friend, family member, or support group can provide motivation and accountability. They can offer encouragement and assistance to keep you sticking to your dietary changes.
- Consider enlisting a buddy to join you on your DASH journey, as having a partner can make the process more enjoyable and effective.

You may provide a strong basis for your DASH Diet action plan by doing these steps. Always keep in mind that leading a heart-healthy lifestyle is a journey, and it's acceptable to go at your own speed.

Stocking Your DASH-Friendly Kitchen

Creating a well-equipped kitchen that supports your DASH Diet journey is a crucial step in ensuring your success. A thoughtfully stocked kitchen can make it easier to prepare healthy, balanced meals that align with the DASH principles. Let's delve deeper into each of these kitchen essentials and explore their significance in your DASH Diet-friendly kitchen:

Fresh Produce

- Fresh fruits & vegetables are the cornerstone of the DASH Diet. They include vital minerals, vitamins, fiber, and antioxidants that promote general health and heart health.
- Make sure you're getting a wide range of nutrients by selecting a number of colorful options. For instance, berries offer antioxidants, while leafy greens like kale, spinach, and collard greens are high in vitamins.

Whole Grains

- Whole grains are an essential component of the DASH Diet, offering a wealth of fiber, vitamins, and minerals. They support the maintenance of energy levels and blood sugar stability throughout the day.
- Eat plenty of whole grains, such as quinoa, brown rice, oats, whole wheat pasta, and whole-grain bread. These staples can be used as the foundation of many DASH-friendly meals.

Lean Proteins

- Lean protein sources are vital for muscle maintenance and overall health. They also aid in making you feel content and full.
- In your kitchen, always have skinless chicken, fish, lean beef or pork chops, tofu, and legumes like beans and lentils on hand. These choices provide a diverse array of options for protein-rich meals.

Low-Fat Dairy

- Dairy products are exceptional sources of calcium and protein. However, it's crucial to select low-fat or fat-free options to minimize saturated fat consumption.
- Keep low-fat or fat-free milk, yogurt, and cheese in your refrigerator. These dairy products can be used in smoothies, cereals, and as a base for healthy sauces.

Healthy Fats

- Incorporating healthy fats is a vital component of a well-rounded diet, supporting heart health while adding satiety and flavor to your meals.
- Use heart-healthy fats like olive oil, canola oil, and avocados for cooking and dressing salads. These fats provide monounsaturated fats, which are beneficial for your heart.

Nuts & Seeds

- Nuts and seeds are abundant in protein, healthy fats, and vital elements including fiber and omega-3 fatty acids.
- Keep a selection of unsalted nuts (e.g., almonds, walnuts) and seeds (e.g., chia seeds, flaxseeds) on hand for snacking and adding texture and flavor to salads, yogurt, or oatmeal.

Herbs and Spices

- Using herbs and spices can help you enhance the taste of your food without using salt. Reducing sodium intake is a fundamental component of the DASH Diet.
- Gather spices like paprika, cumin, and cinnamon, and herbs like basil, rosemary, and thyme. Explore various ingredient combinations to elevate the flavor of your dishes.

Canned Goods

- While fresh produce is ideal, canned vegetables, beans, and tomatoes can be convenient additions to your kitchen.
- Select canned foods that are low in sodium or that don't have any salt to reduce your intake. They can be used in soups, stews, and sauces when fresh options aren't available or for added convenience.

By ensuring your kitchen is stocked with these vital DASH Diet-friendly components, you'll be well-equipped to prepare flavorful and wholesome meals that promote heart health and overall well-being. Planning and organization in the kitchen are key components of successfully following the DASH Diet.

Meal Planning Made Easy: Building Balanced Menus

Creating balanced menus is a fundamental aspect of successfully following the DASH Diet. It requires meticulous preparation and thoughtful assessment of flavor, nutrient balance, and portion sizes. Let's explore each of the steps in detail to help you create DASH-friendly meals that support your heart health and overall well-being:

Use a DASH Meal Planner

- DASH-specific meal planning tools or apps can simplify the process of creating balanced menus. These resources often provide recipes and guidelines tailored to the DASH Diet, making it easier to track your progress and meet your dietary goals.

Focus on Portion Control

- Paying attention to portion sizes is essential to avoid overeating, which can lead to weight gain & increased blood pressure. Use measuring teacups and kitchen scales to become familiar with appropriate portion sizes for different foods.

Balance Macronutrients

- At every meal, try to consume a balanced amount of protein, carbs, and healthy fats. Maintaining this equilibrium provides long-lasting energy and helps to stabilize blood sugar levels.
- Carbohydrates: Include whole grains for complex carbs, such as quinoa, brown rice, and whole wheat bread, along with fruits and vegetables.
- Protein: Include foods high in protein in your diet, such as skinless chicken, fish, tofu, lentils, and low-fat dairy.
- Heart-healthy Fats: To improve flavor and satiety, use nuts, avocado, and olive oil in moderation.

Incorporate a Variety of Foods

- Diversify your diet by including a wide range of foods from all food groups. This ensures that you receive a broad spectrum of vitamins, minerals, and antioxidants.
- Fruits: Incorporate a variety of colorful fruits to provide essential vitamins and fiber.
- Vegetables: To optimize nutrient intake, include a variety of colorful vegetable varieties.
- Whole Grains: For more fiber and nutrients, choose for whole grains like brown rice, oats, and whole wheat pasta.
- Lean Proteins: Rotate between lean protein sources like poultry, fish, legumes, and lean cuts of meat to diversify your protein intake.

Reduce Sodium

- Gradually reduce salt in your recipes to align with the DASH Diet's emphasis on sodium reduction. Excessive sodium consumption may lead to elevated blood pressure levels.
- Incorporate herbs, spices, and salt-free seasonings such as garlic, onion powder, cumin, and lemon juice to enhance the taste of your meals without using salt.

Plan Ahead

- Planning your meals and snacks in advance ensures that you have DASH-friendly options readily available. Using this tactic can help you choose healthier foods even when you're famished and in a rush.
- To ensure you have wholesome meals and snacks throughout the week, think about meal planning and batch cooking on the weekends.

Stay Hydrated

- Remember the significance of maintaining proper hydration. Water can help regulate hunger and avoid overeating, and it is essential for good health in general.
- Reduce your intake of sugary drinks like soda and fruit juices and make water your main beverage of choice.

By following these steps to create balanced menus, you can develop a sustainable and health-conscious approach to eating that aligns with the principles of the DASH Diet. Planning ahead, monitoring portion sizes, and prioritizing nutrient balance and flavor will help you maintain a heart-healthy diet that supports your long-term well-being.

DASH Diet Recipes

Breakfast: Energizing Your Day the DASH Way

1. Avocado Toast with Tomato and Herbs

Preparation time: 10 mins

Cooking time: 0 mins

Servings: 2

Ingredients:

- 2 slices whole-grain bread
- 1 ripe avocado
- 1 tomato, carved
- Fresh basil leaves
- Fresh parsley leaves
- Olive oil for drizzling
- Black pepper as required

Directions:

1. Toast the whole-grain bread slices.
2. While the bread is toasting, mash the ripe avocado in a bowl.
3. Disperse the mashed avocado evenly on the toasted bread slices.
4. Top with carved tomato, fresh basil, and parsley.
5. Spray using olive oil and flavor with black pepper.

Per serving: Calories: 200kcal; Fat: 12g; Carbs: 21g; Protein: 4g; Sodium: 80mg

2. *Banana and Spinach Smoothie*

Preparation time: 5 mins

Cooking time: 0 mins

Servings: 1

Ingredients:

- 1 ripe banana
- 1 teacup fresh spinach leaves
- 1/2 teacup unsweetened almond milk
- 1 tbsp natural almond butter
- 1/2 tsp cinnamon
- Ice cubes (elective)

Directions:

1. Put the entire components inside a mixer.
2. Blend till smooth and creamy.
3. If desired, include ice cubes and blend again.
4. Pour into a glass and relish.

Per serving: Calories: 230kcal; Fat: 8g; Carbs: 39g; Protein: 5g; Sodium: 60mg

3. *Greek Yogurt Parfait with Berries and Nuts*

Preparation time: 5 mins

Cooking time: 0 mins

Servings: 1

Ingredients:

- 1/2 teacup plain Greek yogurt
- 1/4 teacup mixed berries (e.g., strawberries, blueberries, raspberries)
- 1 tbsp severed nuts (e.g., almonds or walnuts)
- 1/2 tsp honey (elective)

Directions:

1. Arrange the Greek yogurt, mixed berries, and chopped almonds in a layer in your glass or bowl.
2. Spray using honey if wanted.
3. Repeat the layering if you have more components.
4. Present chilled.

Per serving: Calories: 250kcal; Fat: 12g; Carbs: 20g; Protein: 15g; Sodium: 60mg

4. *Oatmeal with Sliced Bananas and Almonds*

Preparation time: 5 mins

Cooking time: 5 mins

Servings: 2

Ingredients:

- 1 teacup old-fashioned oats
- 2 teacups water
- 2 ripe bananas, carved
- 2 tbsps severed almonds
- 1/2 tsp cinnamon

Directions:

1. Inside your saucepot, raise water to a boil.
2. Stir in your oats then decrease temp.to simmer.
3. Cook for around 5 minsor 'til the oats are creamy, mixing irregularly.
4. Split your oatmeal into two containers.
5. Top with carved bananas, severed almonds, and a spray of cinnamon.

Per serving: Calories: 250kcal; Fat: 7g; Carbs: 45g; Protein: 6g; Sodium: omg

5. *Scrambled Eggs with Spinach and Feta*

Preparation time: 10 mins

Cooking time: 5 mins

Servings: 2

Ingredients:

- 4 large eggs
- 1 teacup fresh spinach leaves, severed
- 1/4 teacup smashed feta cheese
- Olive oil for cooking
- Freshly ground black pepper

Directions:

1. Inside your container, whisk the eggs till well beaten.
2. Heat your non-stick griddle in a middling temp and include a little olive oil.
3. Include the severed spinach to your griddle then sauté till wilted.
4. Transfer the whisked eggs into the skillet along with the spinach.
5. Cook then stir till the eggs are scrambled and almost set.
6. Spray with smashed feta cheese and black pepper.
7. Continue cooking for an extramin 'til the cheese begins to melt.
8. Present hot.

Per serving: Calories: 220kcal; Fat: 16g; Carbs: 3g; Protein: 15g; Sodium: 280mg

6. *Whole Wheat Pancakes with Fresh Fruit*

Preparation time: 10 mins

Cooking time: 10 mins

Servings: 2

Ingredients:

- 1 teacup whole wheat flour
- 1 tbsp honey
- 1 tsp baking powder
- 1/2 tsp cinnamon
- 1 teacup unsweetened almond milk
- 1 egg
- Fresh fruit (e.g., berries, carved bananas)
- Maple syrup (elective)

Directions:

1. Inside your blending container, blend the whole wheat flour, honey, baking powder, and cinnamon.
2. Inside your distinct container, whisk collectively the almond milk and egg.
3. Put your wet components into the dry components then stir till blended.
4. Warm your non-stick griddle in a middling temp and mildly grease using a small amount of olive oil.
5. Pour 1/4 teacup portions of your pancake batter onto your griddle.
6. Cook the meat till bubbles begin to appear on the surface, turn it, and continue to cook it till the other side is golden brown.
7. Present your pancakes with fresh fruit and a spray of maple syrup if wanted.

Per serving: Calories: 320kcal; Fat: 5g; Carbs: 58g; Protein: 11g; Sodium: 300mg

7. *Vegetable Omelet with a Side of Oranges*

Preparation time: 10 mins

Cooking time: 10 mins

Servings: 2

Ingredients:

- 4 large eggs
- 1/2 teacup cubed bell peppers
- 1/2 teacup cubed onions
- 1/2 teacup carved mushrooms
- 1/2 teacup spinach leaves
- Cooking spray
- 2 oranges, skinned and segmented

Directions:

1. Inside your container, whisk the eggs till well beaten.
2. Heat your non-stick griddle in a middling temp and mildly cover with cooking spray.
3. Include the cubed bell peppers, onions, and mushrooms to your griddle. Sauté till softened.
4. Include the spinach leaves then sauté till wilted.
5. Transfer the whisked eggs into the skillet along with the veggies.
6. Cook, turning the pan to allow the uncooked egg to run below after raising the edges.
7. Once the omelet is mostly set, wrap it in half then cook for an extramin.
8. Present with orange segments on the side.

Per serving: Calories: 230kcal; Fat: 10g; Carbs: 22g; Protein: 15g; Sodium: 150mg

8. *Spinach and Mushroom Breakfast Burrito*
Preparation time: 10 mins
Cooking time: 10 mins
Servings: 2
Ingredients:

- 4 large eggs
- 1 teacup fresh spinach leaves
- 1/2 teacup carved mushrooms
- 1/4 teacup cubed onions
- 2 whole wheat tortillas
- Salsa (elective)

Directions:

1. Inside your container, whisk the eggs till well beaten.
2. Heat your non-stick griddle in a middling temp and mildly cover with cooking spray.
3. Include cubed onions and carved mushrooms to your griddle. Sauté till softened.
4. Include fresh spinach then sauté till wilted.
5. Pour your beaten eggs into your griddle with the vegetables.
6. Cook, stirring, 'til the eggs are scrambled and fully cooked.
7. Warm the whole wheat tortillas in your dry griddle for a couple of secs on all sides.
8. Spoon your egg and vegetable solution onto the tortillas, roll them up, and present.
9. Top with salsa if wanted.

Per serving: Calories: 280kcal; Fat: 12g; Carbs: 25g; Protein: 17g; Sodium: 290mg

9. *Quinoa Porridge with Almond Butter*

Preparation time: 5 mins

Cooking time: 15 mins

Servings: 2

Ingredients:

- 1/2 teacup quinoa, that is washed
- 1 teacup unsweetened almond milk
- 1 tbsp almond butter
- 1/2 tsp vanilla extract
- Fresh berries for topping (elective)

Directions:

1. Inside a saucepot, blend quinoa and almond milk.
2. Boil, then decrease temp to low, cover, then simmer for around 15 minsor 'til quinoa is cooked and the solution densest.
3. Stir in your almond butter and vanilla extract till thoroughly blended.
4. Present in containers, topped with fresh berries if wanted.

Per serving: Calories: 250kcal; Fat: 9g; Carbs: 35g; Protein: 8g; Sodium: 100mg

10. *Berry and Spinach Breakfast Salad*

Preparation time: 10 mins

Cooking time: 0 mins

Servings: 2

Ingredients:

- 2 teacups fresh spinach leaves
- 1 teacup mixed berries (e.g., strawberries, blueberries, raspberries)
- 1/4 teacup severed walnuts
- 2 tbsps balsamic vinaigrette dressing

Directions:

1. Inside your container, blend the fresh spinach leaves, mixed berries, and severed walnuts.
2. Spray using balsamic vinaigrette dressing.
3. Shake to cover evenly and present.

Per serving: Calories: 150kcal; Fat: 11g; Carbs: 12g; Protein: 3g; Sodium: 100mg

11. *Cottage Cheese with Pineapple and Walnuts*

Preparation time: 5 mins

Cooking time: 0 mins

Servings: 2

Ingredients:

- 1 teacup low-fat cottage cheese
- 1 teacup fresh pineapple chunks
- 1/4 teacup severed walnuts
- Honey for drizzling (elective)

Directions:

1. Split your cottage cheese between two containers.
2. Top with fresh pineapple chunks and severed walnuts.
3. Spray using honey if wanted.
4. Present chilled.

Per serving: Calories: 240kcal; Fat: 9g; Carbs: 24g; Protein: 17g; Sodium: 380mg

12. *Overnight Chia Seed Pudding with Berries*

Preparation time: 5 mins (plus overnight chilling)

Cooking time: 0 mins

Servings: 2

Ingredients:

- 1/4 teacup chia seeds
- 1 teacup unsweetened almond milk
- 1/2 tsp vanilla extract
- 1 teacup mixed berries (e.g., strawberries, blueberries, raspberries)
- Honey or maple syrup for drizzling (elective)

Directions:

1. Inside your container, blend chia seeds, almond milk, and vanilla extract.
2. Stir well, cover, then put in the fridge overnight (or for almost 4 hrs).
3. Stir well in the chia pudding early in the morning.
4. Present in containers, topped with mixed berries and a spray of your honey or your maple syrup if wanted.

Per serving: Calories: 200kcal; Fat: 10g; Carbs: 23g; Protein: 6g; Sodium: 100mg

13. Mediterranean Breakfast Bowl

Preparation time: 10 mins

Cooking time: 0 mins

Servings: 2

Ingredients:

- 1 teacup cooked quinoa
- 1/2 teacup cubed cucumber
- 1/2 teacup cubed tomatoes
- 1/4 teacup smashed feta cheese
- 2 tbsps severed Kalamata olives
- 2 tbsps severed fresh parsley
- 2 tsps olive oil
- Lemon juice for drizzling
- Salt and pepper as required

Directions:

1. Inside your container, blend cooked quinoa, cubed cucumber, cubed tomatoes, smashed feta cheese, severed Kalamata olives, and severed fresh parsley.
2. Spray using olive oil and lemon juice.
3. Flavourusing salt and pepper.
4. Shake to mix well and present.

Per serving: Calories: 270kcal; Fat: 13g; Carbs: 29g; Protein: 9g; Sodium: 350mg

14. Almond Flour Banana Muffins

Preparation time: 10 mins

Cooking time: 25 mins

Servings: 12 muffins

Ingredients:

- 2 teacups almond flour
- 2 ripe bananas, mashed
- 3 large eggs
- 1/4 teacup honey
- 1/4 teacup unsweetened almond milk
- 1 tsp baking powder
- 1/2 tsp vanilla extract
- Tweak of salt

Directions:

1. Warm up your oven to 350 deg.F. Use paper liners to line a muffin pan.
2. Inside your blending container, blend almond flour, mashed bananas, eggs, honey, almond milk, baking powder, vanilla extract, and a tweak of salt.
3. Mix till thoroughly blended.
4. Split your batter evenly among your muffin teacups.
5. Bake the muffins for about 25 minutes, or until a toothpick inserted in the center comes out clean.
6. Let the muffins cool down before distributing.

Per serving: Calories: 160kcal; Fat: 11g; Carbs: 12g; Protein: 5g; Sodium: 50mg

15. *Veggie Frittata with Herbs*

Preparation time: 10 mins

Cooking time: 20 mins

Servings: 4

Ingredients:

- 6 big eggs
- 1 teacup severed mixed vegetables (e.g., bell peppers, onions, spinach)
- 2 tbsps severed fresh herbs (e.g., parsley, basil)
- Salt and pepper as required
- Cooking spray
- 1/4 teacup grated low-fat cheese (elective)

Directions:

1. Warm up your oven to 350 deg.F.
2. Inside your container, whisk the eggs and flavour with salt, pepper, and severed herbs.
3. Warm an oven-safe griddle in a middling temp and coat it with cooking spray.
4. Include the severed vegetables to your griddle then sauté till they begin to soften.
5. Evenly drizzle your beaten eggs onto the veggies.
6. Cook for a few mins 'til the edges set.
7. If using cheese, spray it evenly over the frittata.
8. Transfer your skillet to the warmed up oven then bakefor around 10-15 mins, or 'til the frittata is fully set and mildly browned.
9. Slice and present.

Per serving: Calories: 160kcal; Fat: 9g; Carbs: 6g; Protein: 13g; Sodium: 200mg

16. Blueberry and Spinach Smoothie Bowl

Preparation time: 5 mins

Cooking time: 0 mins

Servings: 1

Ingredients:

- 1 teacup fresh spinach leaves
- 1/2 teacup frozen blueberries
- 1/2 ripe banana
- 1/2 teacup unsweetened almond milk
- 1 tbsp chia seeds
- Toppings: Fresh berries, carved banana, severed nuts, honey (elective)

Directions:

1. Put your fresh spinach, almond milk, frozen blueberries, ripe banana, and chia seeds inside a mixer.
2. Blend till smooth and creamy.
3. Pour your smoothie into a container.
4. Top with fresh berries, carved banana, severed nuts, and a spray of honey if wanted.
5. Enjoy with a spoon!

Per serving: Calories: 220kcal; Fat: 7g; Carbs: 35g; Protein: 5g; Sodium: 140mg

17. Sweet Potato Hash with Avocado

Preparation time: 15 mins

Cooking time: 20 mins

Servings: 2

Ingredients:

- 1 large sweet potato, skinned and cubed
- 1/2 red bell pepper, cubed
- 1/2 red onion, cubed
- 1 avocado, carved
- 1 tbsp olive oil
- Salt and pepper as required

Directions:

1. Warm olive oil in your skillet in a med-high temp.
2. Include cubed sweet potato then sauté till it starts to brown and becomes soft (about 10-15 mins).
3. Include cubed red bell pepper and red onion to your griddle and continue to sauté till they are soft.
4. Flavourusing salt and pepper.
5. Present your sweet potato hash with carved avocado on top.

Per serving: Calories: 320kcal; Fat: 19g; Carbs: 36g; Protein: 5g; Sodium: 20mg

18. *Egg White and Veggie Scramble*

Preparation time: 10 mins

Cooking time: 10 mins

Servings: 2

Ingredients:

- 4 large egg whites
- 1/2 teacup cubed mixed vegetables (e.g., bell peppers, tomatoes, zucchini)
- 2 tbsps severed fresh herbs (e.g., chives, cilantro)
- Salt and pepper as required
- Cooking spray

Directions:

1. Inside your container, whisk the egg whites and flavour with salt, pepper, and severed herbs.
2. Heat your non-stick griddle in a middling temp and cover it with cooking spray.
3. Add the diced veggies to the skillet and cook until they begin to soften.
4. Pour your beaten egg whites over the vegetables.
5. Cook, mixing irregularly, 'til the egg whites are fully cooked and scrambled.
6. Present hot.

Per serving: Calories: 60kcal; Fat: 0g; Carbs: 5g; Protein: 12g; Sodium: 220mg

19. *Whole Grain Waffles with Berries*

Preparation time: 10 mins

Cooking time: 10 mins

Servings: 2

Ingredients:

- 2 whole grain waffles (store-bought or homemade)
- 1 teacup mixed berries (e.g., strawberries, blueberries, raspberries)
- 2 tbsps low-fat Greek yogurt
- Maple syrup for drizzling (elective)

Directions:

1. Toast the whole grain waffles using package instructions or your preference.
2. Arrange the heated waffles onto plates for serving.
3. Add some mixed berries and low-fat Greek yogurt over top.
4. Spray using maple syrup if wanted.
5. Present and relish!

Per serving: Calories: 200kcal; Fat: 2g; Carbs: 45g; Protein: 6g; Sodium: 300mg

20. *Spinach and Tomato Breakfast Quesadilla*

Preparation time: 10 mins

Cooking time: 10 mins

Servings: 2

Ingredients:

- 4 whole grain tortillas
- 1 teacup fresh spinach leaves
- 1 large tomato, carved
- 1/2 teacup low-fat shredded cheese
- Cooking spray
- Salsa (elective)

Directions:

1. Lay out two tortillas and top each with fresh spinach, tomato slices, and shredded cheese.
2. To make a sandwich, place another tortilla on top of each one.
3. Warm your non-stick griddle in a middling temp and mildly cover with cooking spray.
4. Gently put the quesadillas in the griddle then cook till they are golden brown then the cheese has dissolved (around 2-3 minson all sides).
5. Present each quesadilla with salsa if desired after slicing it into wedges.

Per serving: Calories: 300kcal; Fat: 10g; Carbs: 40g; Protein: 12g; Sodium: 450mg

21.*Apple Cinnamon Oatmeal*

Preparation time: 5 mins

Cooking time: 10 mins

Servings: 2

Ingredients:

- 1 teacup old-fashioned oats
- 2 teacups unsweetened almond milk
- 1 apple, cubed
- 1/2 tsp ground cinnamon
- 1/4 teacup severed walnuts
- Honey or maple syrup for drizzling (elective)

Directions:

1. Inside a saucepot, blend the oats, almond milk, cubed apple, and ground cinnamon.
2. Raise to a simmer in a middling temp then cook, mixing irregularly, 'til the oats are soft and creamy (around 10 mins).
3. Split your oatmeal into two containers.
4. Top with severed walnuts then spray with honey or maple syrup if wanted.

Per serving: Calories: 300kcal; Fat: 12g; Carbs: 42g; Protein: 7g; Sodium: 170mg

22. *Breakfast Quinoa with Pecans and Raisins*

Preparation time: 5 mins

Cooking time: 15 mins

Servings: 2

Ingredients:

- 1 teacup cooked quinoa
- 1/4 teacup severed pecans
- 1/4 teacup raisins
- 1/2 tsp ground cinnamon
- 1 tbsp honey
- Low-fat milk or almond milk for drizzling (elective)

Directions:

1. Inside your container, blend the cooked quinoa, severed pecans, raisins, ground cinnamon, and honey.
2. Mix well.
3. Present in containers with a spray of low-fat milk or almond milk if wanted.

Per serving: Calories: 280kcal; Fat: 10g; Carbs: 45g; Protein: 5g; Sodium: 5mg

23. *Breakfast Tacos with Salsa*

Preparation time: 10 mins

Cooking time: 10 mins

Servings: 2

Ingredients:

- 4 small whole wheat tortillas
- 4 large eggs
- 1/2 teacup cubed bell peppers
- 1/2 teacup cubed onions
- Cooking spray
- Salsa (homemade or store-bought)

Directions:

1. Warm your non-stick griddle in a middling temp and coat it with cooking spray.
2. Bring cubed bell peppers and onions to your griddle then sauté till softened.
3. Inside your container, beat the eggs.
4. Pour your beaten eggs into your griddle with the sautéed vegetables.
5. Cook, mixing irregularly, 'til the eggs are scrambled and fully cooked.
6. Warm the tortillas in your dry griddle for a couple of secs on all sides.
7. Split your scrambled eggs and vegetable solution evenly among the tortillas.
8. Top with salsa.
9. Wrap the tortillas and present.

Per serving: Calories: 300kcal; Fat: 11g; Carbs: 30g; Protein: 18g; Sodium: 350mg

24. *Banana Walnut Muffins*

Preparation time: 15 mins

Cooking time: 20 mins

Servings: 12 muffins

Ingredients:

- 2 teacups whole wheat flour
- 1 tsp baking powder
- 1/2 tsp baking soda
- 1/2 tsp ground cinnamon
- 2 ripe bananas, mashed
- 1/2 teacup unsweetened applesauce
- 1/4 teacup honey
- 2 large eggs
- 1/2 teacup severed walnuts

Directions:

1. Warm up your oven to 350 deg.F. Use paper liners to line a muffin pan.
2. Combine ground cinnamon, baking soda, baking powder, and whole wheat flour in your container.
3. In another bowl, mix mashed bananas, applesauce, honey, and eggs till thoroughly blended.
4. Put your wet components into the dry components then stir till blended.
5. Wrap in the severed walnuts.
6. Split your batter evenly among your muffin teacups.
7. Bake for around 20 minsor 'til a toothpick immersed into your muffin comes out clean.
8. Allow the muffins to cool before serving.

Per serving: Calories: 160kcal; Fat: 5g; Carbs: 27g; Protein: 4g; Sodium: 90mg

Lunch: Quick and Nutrient-Rich Midday Meals

25. *Spinach and Chickpea Salad with Olive Oil Dressing*

Preparation time: 10 mins

Cooking time: 0 mins

Servings: 2

Ingredients:

- 4 teacups fresh spinach leaves
- 1 tin (15 oz.) chickpeas, that is drained and washed
- 1/4 teacup carved red onion
- 1/4 teacup carved cucumber
- 1/4 teacup cherry tomatoes, divided
- 2 tbsps extra-virgin olive oil
- 1 tbsp balsamic vinegar
- Salt and pepper as required

Directions:

1. Inside your big container, blend fresh spinach, chickpeas, red onion, cucumber, and cherry tomatoes.
2. In your separate small container, whisk collectively olive oil and balsamic vinegar to form your dressing.
3. Transfer the dressing over the salad and shake to cover.
4. Flavourusing salt and pepper as required.
5. Split into two containers and present.

Per serving: Calories: 350kcal; Fat: 17g; Carbs: 42g; Protein: 11g; Sodium: 450mg

26. *Quinoa and Black Bean Bowl with Avocado*

Preparation time: 15 mins

Cooking time: 15 mins

Servings: 2

Ingredients:

- 1 teacup cooked quinoa
- 1 tin (15 oz.) black beans, that is drained and washed
- 1/2 teacup cubed red bell pepper
- 1/2 teacup cubed red onion
- 1 avocado, carved
- Juice of 1 lime
- Fresh cilantro leaves for garnish
- Salt and pepper as required

Directions:

1. Inside your big container, blend cooked quinoa, black beans, cubed red bell pepper, and cubed red onion.
2. Spray using lime juice and toss to blend.
3. Flavourusing salt and pepper.
4. Split into two containers and top with carved avocado and fresh cilantro leaves.
5. Present.

Per serving: Calories: 350kcal; Fat: 14g; Carbs: 50g; Protein: 12g; Sodium: 400mg

27. *Greek Salad with Grilled Chicken*

Preparation time: 15 mins

Cooking time: 15 mins

Servings: 2

Ingredients:

- 2 boneless, skinless chicken breasts
- 4 teacups mixed salad greens
- 1/2 teacup cherry tomatoes, divided
- 1/4 teacup carved cucumber
- 1/4 teacup carved red onion
- 1/4 teacup Kalamata olives, eroded
- 1/4 teacups mashed feta cheese
- Greek salad dressing (store-bought or homemade)

Directions:

1. Flavour your chicken breasts using salt and pepper.
2. Grill the chicken inside a med-high temp till cooked through (around 6-8 minson all sides).
3. Slice the grilled chicken into strips.
4. Combine mixed salad greens, cucumber, red onion, cherry tomatoes, Kalamata olives, and crumbled feta cheese in a large container.
5. Top with grilled chicken strips.
6. Spray using Greek salad dressing.
7. Shake to cover and present.

Per serving: Calories: 320kcal; Fat: 12g; Carbs: 15g; Protein: 35g; Sodium: 780mg

28. *Turkey and Avocado Wrap on Whole Wheat Tortilla*

Preparation time: 10 mins

Cooking time: 0 mins

Servings: 2

Ingredients:

- 2 whole wheat tortillas
- 8 slices of lean turkey breast
- 1 avocado, carved
- 1 teacup mixed salad greens
- 2 tbsps Greek yogurt (or low-fat mayo)
- 1 tsp Dijon mustard
- Salt and pepper as required

Directions:

1. Inside your small container, mix Greek yogurt (or mayo) and Dijon mustard to form the dressing.
2. Lay out two whole wheat tortillas.
3. Disperse the dressing evenly on each tortilla.
4. Layer with lean turkey breast slices, avocado slices, and mixed salad greens.
5. Flavourusing salt and pepper as required.
6. Roll up the tortillas firmly, slice in half if wanted, and present.

Per serving: Calories: 350kcal; Fat: 15g; Carbs: 31g; Protein: 23g; Sodium: 480mg

29. *Spinach and Mushroom Quesadilla*

Preparation time: 15 mins

Cooking time: 10 mins

Servings: 2

Ingredients:

- 4 whole wheat tortillas
- 2 teacups fresh spinach leaves
- 1 teacup carved mushrooms
- 1/2 teacup shredded low-fat mozzarella cheese
- 1/4 teacup cubed red onion
- Cooking spray
- Salsa (elective)

Directions:

1. Warm your non-stick griddle in a middling temp and mildly cover with cooking spray.
2. Include carved mushrooms and cubed red onion to your griddle then sauté till softened.
3. Lay out two tortillas and spray each with shredded mozzarella cheese.
4. Top with fresh spinach and the sautéed mushrooms and onions.

5. To make a sandwich, place another tortilla on top of each one.
6. Carefully transfer the quesadillas to your griddle then cook till they are golden brown then the cheese has dissolved (around 2-3 minson all sides).
7. Present each quesadilla with salsa if desired after slicing it into wedges.

Per serving: Calories: 350kcal; Fat: 10g; Carbs: 48g; Protein: 18g; Sodium: 500mg

30. *Tuna Salad with Mixed Greens*

Preparation time: 10 mins

Cooking time: 0 mins

Servings: 2

Ingredients:

- 2 tins (5 oz. each) of water-packed tuna, drained
- 4 teacups mixed salad greens
- 1/2 teacup cherry tomatoes, divided
- 1/4 teacup cubed cucumber
- 1/4 teacup cubed bell peppers
- 2 tbsps lemon juice
- 2 tbsps olive oil
- Salt and pepper as required

Directions:

1. Inside your container, blend drained tuna, mixed salad greens, cherry tomatoes, cubed cucumber, and cubed bell peppers.
2. Inside your distinct small container, whisk collectively lemon juice and olive oil to create your dressing.
3. Transfer the dressing over the salad and shake to cover.
4. Flavourusing salt and pepper as required.
5. Split into two containers and present.

Per serving: Calories: 270kcal; Fat: 12g; Carbs: 8g; Protein: 32g; Sodium: 500mg

31. *Hummus and Veggie Wrap*

Preparation time: 10 mins

Cooking time: 0 mins

Servings: 2

Ingredients:

- 2 whole wheat tortillas
- 1/2 teacup hummus (store-bought or homemade)
- 1 teacup mixed salad greens
- 1/2 teacup cubed tomatoes
- 1/2 teacup carved cucumbers

- 1/4 teacup carved red onion
- Salt and pepper as required

Directions:

1. Lay out two whole wheat tortillas.
2. Disperse 1/4 teacup of hummus evenly on each tortilla.
3. Top with mixed salad greens, cubed tomatoes, carved cucumbers, and carved red onion.
4. Flavourusing salt and pepper as required.
5. Roll up the tortillas firmly, slice in half if wanted, and present.

Per serving: Calories: 320kcal; Fat: 16g; Carbs: 36g; Protein: 11g; Sodium: 650mg

32. *Spinach and Strawberry Salad with Balsamic Vinaigrette*

Preparation time: 10 mins

Cooking time: 0 mins

Servings: 2

Ingredients:

- 4 teacups fresh spinach leaves
- 1 teacup carved strawberries
- 1/4 teacup smashed feta cheese
- 2 tbsps severed pecans or walnuts
- Balsamic vinaigrette dressing (store-bought or homemade)

Directions:

1. Inside your big container, blend fresh spinach, carved strawberries, smashed feta cheese, and severed pecans or walnuts.
2. Spray using balsamic vinaigrette dressing.
3. Shake to cover and present.

Per serving: Calories: 220kcal; Fat: 14g; Carbs: 18g; Protein: 6g; Sodium: 340mg

33. *Caprese Sandwich with Pesto*

Preparation time: 10 mins

Cooking time: 0 mins

Servings: 2

Ingredients:

- 4 slices whole wheat bread
- 2 large tomatoes, carved
- 4 oz. fresh mozzarella cheese, carved
- 2 tbsps basil pesto (store-bought or homemade)
- Fresh basil leaves for garnish (elective)

Directions:

1. Disperse 1 tbsp of basil pesto on every slice of whole wheat bread.
2. On two slices of bread, layer tomato slices and fresh mozzarella cheese slices.
3. Top with fresh basil leaves if wanted.
4. Put your remaining slices of bread on top to form sandwiches.
5. Slice in half if wanted and present.

Per serving: Calories: 370kcal; Fat: 18g; Carbs: 37g; Protein: 16g; Sodium: 500mg

34. *Mixed Bean Salad with Herbs*

Preparation time: 10 mins

Cooking time: 0 mins

Servings: 4

Ingredients:

- 2 teacups mixed beans (e.g., kidney beans, black beans, chickpeas), canned and drained
- 1 teacup cubed bell peppers (any color)
- 1/2 teacup cubed red onion
- 1/2 teacup severed fresh parsley
- 2 tbsps extra-virgin olive oil
- 2 tbsps balsamic vinegar
- Salt and pepper as required

Directions:

1. Inside your big container, blend mixed beans, cubed bell peppers, cubed red onion, and severed fresh parsley.
2. Inside your distinct small container, whisk collectively olive oil and balsamic vinegar to form your dressing.
3. Transfer the dressing over the salad and shake to cover.
4. Flavourusing salt and pepper as required.
5. Present chilled.

Per serving: Calories: 210kcal; Fat: 7g; Carbs: 31g; Protein: 9g; Sodium: 250mg

35. *Grilled Salmon Salad with Lemon-Dill Dressing*

Preparation time: 15 mins

Cooking time: 10 mins

Servings: 2

Ingredients:

- 2 salmon fillets
- 4 teacups mixed salad greens
- 1/2 teacup cherry tomatoes, divided
- 1/4 teacup carved cucumber

- 1/4 teacup carved red onion
- For the Lemon-Dill Dressing:
- 2 tbsps fresh lemon juice
- 1 tbsp extra-virgin olive oil
- 1 tsp fresh dill, severed
- Salt and pepper as required

Directions:

1. Flavour your salmon fillets using salt and pepper.
2. Grill the salmon inside a med-high temp till cooked through (around 4-5 minson all sides).
3. Inside your big container, blend mixed salad greens, carved cucumber, cherry tomatoes, and carved red onion.
4. Inside your small container, whisk collectively fresh lemon juice, extra-virgin olive oil, fresh dill, salt, and pepper to form the dressing.
5. Top the salad with the grilled salmon and drizzle with the Lemon-Dill Dressing.
6. Present.

Per serving: Calories: 330kcal; Fat: 18g; Carbs: 11g; Protein: 30g; Sodium: 130mg

36. *Vegetable Stir-Fry with Tofu*

Preparation time: 15 mins

Cooking time: 15 mins

Servings: 4

Ingredients:

- 14 oz. firm tofu, cubed
- 2 teacups mixed vegetables (e.g., broccoli, bell peppers, snap peas), carved
- 1/4 teacup low-sodium soy sauce
- 2 pieces garlic, crushed
- 1 tbsp fresh ginger, grated
- 2 tbsps sesame oil
- 1 tbsp cornstarch mixed using 2 tbsps water
- Cooked brown rice for serving

Directions:

1. In your wok or large skillet, heat sesame oil in a med-high temp.
2. Include tofu cubes then stir-fry till mildly browned.
3. Take out tofu from the pan then put away.
4. Inside the similar pot, include mixed vegetables then stir-fry for 3-4 mins 'tilsoft.
5. Inside your small container, whisk collectively low-sodium soy sauce, crushed garlic, and grated ginger.
6. Pour your sauce over the vegetables and include the cornstarch-water solution.
7. Stir till the sauce denses.

8. Return the tofu to the pan then stir till heated through.
9. Present over cooked brown rice.

Per serving: Calories: 180kcal; Fat: 9g; Carbs: 11g; Protein: 15g; Sodium: 480mg

37. *Quinoa and Spinach Stuffed Peppers*

Preparation time: 20 mins

Cooking time: 40 mins

Servings: 4

Ingredients:

- 4 bell peppers, any color
- 1 teacup quinoa, cooked
- 2 teacups fresh spinach leaves, severed
- 1 tin (15 oz.) cubed tomatoes, drained
- 1/2 teacup low-sodium vegetable broth
- 1/2 teacup smashed feta cheese
- 2 tbsps fresh basil, severed
- Salt and pepper as required

Directions:

1. Warm up your oven to 375 deg.F.
2. Remove the bell peppers' tops, cut them in half lengthwise, and throw away the seeds and membranes.
3. Inside your big container, blend cooked quinoa, severed fresh spinach, cubed tomatoes, vegetable broth, smashed feta cheese, severed fresh basil, salt, and pepper.
4. Place a portion of the quinoa and spinach solution inside of all bell peppers.
5. Put your stuffed peppers in your baking dish and cover using foil.
6. Bake for around 30-35 minsor 'til the peppers are soft.
7. Take out foil then bake for an extra 5 mins 'til the tops are mildly browned.
8. Present.

Per serving: Calories: 250kcal; Fat: 7g; Carbs: 38g; Protein: 11g; Sodium: 480mg

38. *Chicken and Vegetable Kabobs*

Preparation time: 15 mins

Cooking time: 15 mins

Servings: 4

Ingredients:

- 1 lb. boneless, skinless chicken breasts, that is cut into chunks
- 2 teacups mixed vegetables (e.g., bell peppers, zucchini, cherry tomatoes), that is cut into chunks
- 2 tbsps olive oil
- 1 tbsp lemon juice
- 2 pieces garlic, crushed
- 1 tsp dried oregano
- Salt and pepper as required
- Skewers (metal or wooden, soaked in water)

Directions:

1. Inside your container, whisk collectively olive oil, crushed garlic, dried oregano, lemon juice, salt, and pepper to form the marinade.
2. Alternating between chicken and veggies, thread mixed vegetables and chicken onto skewers.
3. Put your skewers in a shallow dish and brush with the marinade.
4. Warm up your grill to med-high temp.
5. Grill the kabobs for around 6-7 minson all sides or 'til the chicken is cooked through and the vegetables are soft.
6. Present hot.

Per serving: Calories: 230kcal; Fat: 10g; Carbs: 8g; Protein: 25g; Sodium: 120mg

39. *Mediterranean Quinoa Salad*

Preparation time: 15 mins

Cooking time: 15 mins

Servings: 4

Ingredients:

- 1 teacup quinoa, that is washed then cooked
- 1 teacup cubed cucumber
- 1 teacup cherry tomatoes, divided
- 1/2 teacup cubed red onion
- 1/2 teacup Kalamata olives, that is eroded and carved
- 1/2 teacup smashed feta cheese
- 1/4 teacup fresh parsley, severed
- For the Dressing:

- 3 tbsps extra-virgin olive oil
- 2 tbsps lemon juice
- 2 pieces garlic, crushed
- Salt and pepper as required

Directions:

1. Inside your big container, blend cooked quinoa, cubed cucumber, cherry tomatoes, cubed red onion, Kalamata olives, smashed feta cheese, and severed fresh parsley.
2. Inside your small container, whisk collectively extra-virgin olive oil, salt, lemon juice, crushed garlic, and pepper to form the dressing.
3. Transfer the dressing over the salad and shake to cover.
4. Present chilled.

Per serving: Calories: 350kcal; Fat: 20g; Carbs: 35g; Protein: 10g; Sodium: 450mg

40. *Turkey and Vegetable Stir-Fry*

Preparation time: 15 mins

Cooking time: 15 mins

Servings: 4

Ingredients:

- 1 lb. lean ground turkey
- 4 teacups mixed vegetables (e.g., bell peppers, broccoli, snap peas), carved
- 2 pieces garlic, crushed
- 1 tbsp fresh ginger, grated
- 2 tbsps low-sodium soy sauce
- 1 tbsp hoisin sauce
- 1 tbsp sesame oil
- 2 tbsps severed scallions
- Cooked brown rice for serving

Directions:

1. Inside your big griddle or wok, cook ground turkey in a med-high temp till browned then cooked through.
2. Take out the cooked turkey from the griddle and put away.
3. Inside the similar griddle, include mixed vegetables, crushed garlic, and grated ginger. Stir-fry for around 5 mins 'til the vegetables are soft-crisp.
4. Return the cooked turkey to your griddle.
5. Inside your small container, whisk collectively low-sodium soy sauce, hoisin sauce, and sesame oil.
6. Cover the turkey and veggies with your sauce. Stir to coat evenly then cook for an extra 2-3 mins.
7. Garnish using severed scallions.

8. Present over cooked brown rice.

Per serving: Calories: 250kcal; Fat: 9g; Carbs: 15g; Protein: 26g; Sodium: 380mg

41.*Chickpea and Spinach Curry*
Preparation time: 15 mins
Cooking time: 20 mins
Servings: 4
Ingredients:

- 2 tins (15 oz. each) chickpeas, that is drained and washed
- 1 onion, finely severed
- 2 pieces garlic, crushed
- 1-inch piece of fresh ginger, grated
- 1 tin (14 oz.) cubed tomatoes
- 2 teacups fresh spinach leaves
- 1 tbsp olive oil
- 1 tbsp curry powder
- 1/2 tsp ground turmeric
- Salt and pepper as required

Directions:

1. Warm olive oil inside your big griddle in a middling temp.
2. Include finely severed onion then cook till translucent.
3. Stir in your crushed garlic and grated ginger; cook for an extramin.
4. Include curry powder and ground turmeric; cook for 1-2 mins 'til fragrant.
5. Pour in cubed tomatoes and chickpeas. Flavourusing salt and pepper.
6. Simmer for around 10 mins, mixing irregularly.
7. Stir in fresh spinach leaves then cook till wilted.
8. Present warm.

Per serving: Calories: 280kcal; Fat: 5g; Carbs: 47g; Protein: 13g; Sodium: 590mg

42. *Spinach and Feta Stuffed Chicken Breast*
Preparation time: 15 mins
Cooking time: 25 mins
Servings: 4
Ingredients:

- 4 boneless, skinless chicken breasts
- 2 teacups fresh spinach leaves
- 1/2 teacup smashed feta cheese
- 2 pieces garlic, crushed

- Salt and pepper as required
- Olive oil for cooking

Directions:

1. Warm up your oven to 375 deg.F.
2. Butterfly each chicken breast by cutting a slit horizontally, creating a pocket.
3. Inside your container, blend fresh spinach leaves, smashed feta cheese, crushed garlic, salt, and pepper.
4. Stuff every chicken breast using the spinach and feta solution.
5. In an oven-safe skillet over medium-high heat, preheat the olive oil.
6. Brown the stuffed chicken breasts for around 2-3 mins on all sides.
7. Transfer your griddle to the warmed up oven then bake for around 15-20 minsor 'til the chicken is cooked through.
8. Present warm.

Per serving: Calories: 220kcal; Fat: 9g; Carbs: 2g; Protein: 32g; Sodium: 370mg

43. *Zucchini Noodles with Pesto*

Preparation time: 10 mins

Cooking time: 5 mins

Servings: 4

Ingredients:

- 4 medium zucchinis, spiralized into noodles
- 1/2 teacup basil pesto (store-bought or homemade)
- 1/4 teacup grated Parmesan cheese
- Cherry tomatoes for garnish (elective)

Directions:

1. Inside your big griddle, warm a bit of olive oil in a middling temp.
2. Include the zucchini noodles then sauté for around 3-4 mins 'til they are just soft.
3. Take out the griddle from heat.
4. Stir in basil pesto and grated Parmesan cheese till the noodles are coated evenly.
5. Garnish using cherry tomatoes if wanted.
6. Present hot.

Per serving: Calories: 280kcal; Fat: 25g; Carbs: 7g; Protein: 7g; Sodium: 440mg

44. *Avocado and Black Bean Salad*

Preparation time: 15 mins

Cooking time: 0 mins

Servings: 4

Ingredients:

- 2 avocados, cubed
- 1 tin (15 oz.) black beans, that is drained and washed
- 1 teacup corn kernels
- 1/2 teacup cubed red onion
- 1/4 teacup severed fresh cilantro
- 2 tbsps fresh lime juice
- 2 tbsps extra-virgin olive oil
- Salt and pepper as required

Directions:

1. Inside your big container, blend cubed avocados, black beans, corn kernels, cubed red onion, and severed fresh cilantro.
2. Inside your small container, whisk collectively extra-virgin olive oil, salt, fresh lime juice, and pepper to form your dressing.
3. Transfer the dressing over the salad and toss gently to cover.
4. Present chilled.

Per serving: Calories: 270kcal; Fat: 15g; Carbs: 30g; Protein: 7g; Sodium: 240mg

45. *Turkey and Vegetable Lettuce Wraps*

Preparation time: 15 mins

Cooking time: 15 mins

Servings: 4

Ingredients:

- 1 lb. lean ground turkey
- 1 teacup mixed bell peppers, cubed
- 1/2 teacup cubed carrots
- 1/2 teacup cubed zucchini
- 2 pieces garlic, crushed
- 2 tbsps low-sodium soy sauce
- 1 tbsp hoisin sauce
- 1 tsp sesame oil
- Iceberg or butter lettuce leaves for wrapping

Directions:

1. Inside your big griddle, cook lean ground turkey in a med-high temp till browned then cooked through.

2. Take out the cooked turkey from the griddle and put away.

3. Inside the similar griddle, include mixed bell peppers, cubed carrots, cubed zucchini, and crushed garlic. Sauté for around 5 mins 'til the vegetables are soft-crisp.

4. Return the cooked turkey to your griddle.

5. Inside your small container, whisk collectively low-sodium soy sauce, hoisin sauce, and sesame oil.

6. Cover the turkey and veggies with your sauce. Stir to coat evenly then cook for an extra 2-3 mins.

7. Present your turkey and vegetable solution in lettuce leaves.

Per serving: Calories: 200kcal; Fat: 7g; Carbs: 10g; Protein: 23g; Sodium: 380mg

46. *Spinach and Lentil Salad with Citrus Dressing*

Preparation time: 15 mins

Cooking time: 20 mins

Servings: 4

Ingredients:

- 1 teacup green or brown lentils, that is washed
- 4 teacups fresh spinach leaves
- 1/2 teacup cherry tomatoes, divided
- 1/4 teacup cubed red onion
- 1/4 teacup severed fresh parsley
- For the Citrus Dressing:
- Juice of 1 orange
- Juice of 1 lemon
- 2 tbsps extra-virgin olive oil
- 1 tsp Dijon mustard
- Salt and pepper as required

Directions:

1. Inside a saucepot, blend washed lentils with sufficient water to cover them by about an inch.

2. Boil, then decrease temp.to simmer then cook for around 20 mins 'til lentils are soft but not mushy.

3. After draining any excess water, let the lentils to cool.

4. Inside your big container, blend cooked lentils, fresh spinach leaves, cherry tomatoes, cubed red onion, and severed fresh parsley.

5. Inside your distinct small container, whisk collectively orange juice, lemon juice, extra-virgin olive oil, Dijon mustard, salt, and pepper to form the dressing.

6. Transfer the dressing over the salad and shake to cover.

7. Present chilled.

Per serving: Calories: 240kcal; Fat: 7g; Carbs: 34g; Protein: 13g; Sodium: 90mg

47. *Cucumber and Tomato Salad with Olive Oil*

Preparation time: 10 mins

Cooking time: 0 mins

Servings: 4

Ingredients:

- 2 cucumbers, carved
- 2 teacups cherry tomatoes, divided
- 1/4 teacup red onion, thinly carved
- 2 tbsps extra-virgin olive oil
- 2 tbsps fresh lemon juice
- 2 tbsps fresh dill, severed
- Salt and pepper as required

Directions:

1. Inside your big container, blend cucumber slices, cherry tomatoes, and thinly carved red onion.
2. Inside your small container, whisk collectively extra-virgin olive oil, fresh lemon juice, severed fresh dill, salt, and pepper to form your dressing.
3. Pour the dressing over the salad, then give it a light shake to distribute it evenly.
4. Present chilled.

Per serving: Calories: 90kcal; Fat: 7g; Carbs: 7g; Protein: 1g; Sodium: 10mg

48. *Spinach and Quinoa Bowl with Feta*

Preparation time: 15 mins

Cooking time: 15 mins

Servings: 4

Ingredients:

- 1 teacup quinoa, that is washed then cooked
- 4 teacups fresh spinach leaves
- 1/2 teacup smashed feta cheese
- 1/4 teacup severed Kalamata olives
- 2 tbsps extra-virgin olive oil
- 2 tbsps balsamic vinegar
- Salt and pepper as required

Directions:

1. Inside your big container, blend cooked quinoa, fresh spinach leaves, smashed feta cheese, and severed Kalamata olives.
2. Inside your small container, whisk collectively extra-virgin olive oil, salt, balsamic vinegar, and pepper to form the dressing.
3. Transfer the dressing over the bowl and toss carefully to coat.
4. Present.

Per serving: Calories: 290kcal; Fat: 17g; Carbs: 27g; Protein: 9g; Sodium: 400mg

Dinner: Savory, Satisfying Dishes for Every Palate

49. *Baked Salmon with Lemon and Dill*

Preparation time: 10 mins

Cooking time: 15 mins

Servings: 4

Ingredients:

- 4 salmon fillets
- Zest and juice of 1 lemon
- 2 tbsps fresh dill, severed
- 2 pieces garlic, crushed
- Salt and pepper as required
- Olive oil for drizzling

Directions:

1. Warm up your oven to 375 deg.F.
2. Put your salmon fillets on your baking sheet covered with parchment paper.
3. Inside your small container, blend lemon zest, lemon juice, severed fresh dill, crushed garlic, salt, and pepper.
4. Spray the lemon-dill solution over the salmon fillets.
5. Spray using a bit of olive oil.
6. Bake for around 15 minsor 'til the salmon flakes simply using a fork.
7. Present warm.

Per serving: Calories: 250kcal; Fat: 11g; Carbs: 2g; Protein: 33g; Sodium: 90mg

50. *Grilled Chicken with Spinach and Tomato Salsa*

Preparation time: 15 mins

Cooking time: 15 mins

Servings: 4

Ingredients:

- 4 boneless, skinless chicken breasts
- 4 teacups fresh spinach leaves
- 2 teacups cherry tomatoes, divided
- 1/4 teacup cubed red onion
- 2 pieces garlic, crushed
- 2 tbsps balsamic vinegar
- 2 tbsps extra-virgin olive oil
- Salt and pepper as required

Directions:

1. Flavour your chicken breasts using salt and pepper.

2. Warm up your grill to med-high temp.
3. Grill the chicken for around 6-7 minson all sides or 'til cooked through.
4. Inside your big container, blend fresh spinach leaves, cherry tomatoes, cubed red onion, and crushed garlic.
5. Inside your distinct small container, whisk collectively balsamic vinegar and extra-virgin olive oil to form your dressing.
6. Transfer the dressing across the salad and shake to cover.
7. Present grilled chicken on top of the spinach and tomato salad.

Per serving: Calories: 280kcal; Fat: 11g; Carbs: 10g; Protein: 34g; Sodium: 150mg

51. *Spaghetti Squash with Tomato and Basil Sauce*
Preparation time: 15 mins
Cooking time: 40 mins
Servings: 4
Ingredients:

- 1 large spaghetti squash, divided and seeded
- 2 teacups cubed tomatoes (canned or fresh)
- 1/4 teacup severed fresh basil
- 2 pieces garlic, crushed
- 2 tbsps extra-virgin olive oil
- Salt and pepper as required
- Grated Parmesan cheese for garnish (elective)

Directions:

1. Warm up your oven to 375 deg.F.
2. Put your spaghetti squash halves cut side down on your baking sheet.
3. Roast in the oven for around 35-40 mins 'til the squash is soft and can be easily scraped into "noodles" using a fork.
4. As you roast your squash, make the sauce. Inside a saucepot, heat extra-virgin olive oil inside a middling temp include crushed garlic then sauté for 1-2 mins 'til fragrant.
5. Stir in cubed tomatoes and severed fresh basil. Cook for 5-10 mins, allowing the flavors to meld. Flavourusing salt and pepper.
6. Scrape the roasted spaghetti squash into "noodles" using a fork.
7. Present your squash topped with the tomato and basil sauce.
8. Garnish using grated Parmesan cheese if wanted.

Per serving: Calories: 110kcal; Fat: 7g; Carbs: 12g; Protein: 2g; Sodium: 110mg

52. *Lentil and Spinach Curry*

Preparation time: 15 mins

Cooking time: 25 mins

Servings: 4

Ingredients:

- 1 teacup dry green or brown lentils, that is washed
- 4 teacups fresh spinach leaves
- 1 tin (14 oz.) cubed tomatoes
- 1 onion, finely severed
- 2 pieces garlic, crushed
- 1" piece of fresh ginger, grated
- 2 tbsps curry powder
- 1 tbsp olive oil
- Salt and pepper as required

Directions:

1. Inside a saucepot, blend washed lentils with sufficient water to cover them by about an inch.
2. Boil, then decrease temp.to simmer then cook for around 20-25 mins 'til lentils are soft but not mushy. Drain any extra water.
3. Inside your big griddle, warm olive oil in a middling temp.
4. Include finely severed onion then cook till translucent.
5. Add the curry powder, grated ginger, and crushed garlic. Cook for 1-2 mins 'til fragrant.
6. Pour in cubed tomatoes then cooked lentils. Flavourusing salt and pepper.
7. Simmer for around 10 mins, mixing irregularly.
8. Stir in fresh spinach leaves then cook till wilted.
9. Present hot.

Per serving: Calories: 250kcal; Fat: 3g; Carbs: 44g; Protein: 14g; Sodium: 480mg

53. *Grilled Shrimp with Avocado Salsa*

Preparation time: 15 mins

Cooking time: 5 mins

Servings: 4

Ingredients:

- 1 lb. large shrimp, skinned and deveined
- 2 avocados, cubed
- 1 teacup cubed tomatoes
- 1/4 teacup cubed red onion
- 1/4 teacup severed fresh cilantro
- 2 tbsps fresh lime juice
- 2 tbsps extra-virgin olive oil
- Salt and pepper as required

Directions:

1. Warm up your grill to med-high temp.
2. Flavour your shrimp using salt and pepper.
3. Grill the shrimp for around 2-3 minson all sides or 'til they turn pink and opaque.
4. Inside your big container, blend cubed avocados, cubed tomatoes, cubed red onion, severed fresh cilantro, fresh lime juice, and extra-virgin olive oil.
5. Add some salt and pepper to your avocado salsa to taste it.
6. Present grilled shrimp on top of the avocado salsa.

Per serving: Calories: 300kcal; Fat: 20g; Carbs: 15g; Protein: 18g; Sodium: 260mg

54. *Quinoa-Stuffed Bell Peppers*

Preparation time: 20 mins

Cooking time: 45 mins

Servings: 4

Ingredients:

- 4 bell peppers, any color
- 1 teacup quinoa, that is washed then cooked
- 1 teacup black beans, canned and drained
- 1 teacup cubed tomatoes (canned or fresh)
- 1/2 teacup corn kernels
- 1/2 teacup cubed red onion
- 2 pieces garlic, crushed
- 1 tsp ground cumin
- 1/2 tsp chili powder
- Salt and pepper as required
- 1/2 teacup shredded cheddar cheese (elective)

Directions:

1. Warm up your oven to 375 deg.F.
2. Remove the seeds and membranes from your bell peppers by cutting off the tops.
3. Inside your big container, blend cooked quinoa, black beans, cubed tomatoes, corn kernels, cubed red onion, crushed garlic, ground cumin, chili powder, salt, and pepper.
4. Fill each bell pepper with the veggie and quinoa mixture.
5. Garnish each stuffed pepper with shredded cheddar cheese, if you'd like.
6. Put your stuffed peppers in your baking dish and cover using foil.
7. Bake for around 30-35 minsor 'til the peppers are soft.
8. Take out foil then bake for an extra 5 mins 'til the cheese is dissolved& bubbly (if using).
9. Present warm.

Per serving: Calories: 280kcal; Fat: 2g; Carbs: 56g; Protein: 12g; Sodium: 330mg

55. *Vegetable Stir-Fry with Brown Rice*

Preparation time: 15 mins

Cooking time: 15 mins

Servings: 4

Ingredients:

- 2 teacups cooked brown rice
- 2 teacups mixed vegetables (e.g., broccoli, bell peppers, carrots), carved
- 1 teacup snap peas, clipped
- 1/2 teacup carved mushrooms
- 1/4 teacup low-sodium soy sauce

- 2 pieces garlic, crushed
- 1 tbsp fresh ginger, grated
- 1 tbsp olive oil
- 1 tsp cornstarch mixed using 2 tbsps water

Directions:

1. In your wok or large skillet, warm olive oil in a med-high temp.
2. Include mixed vegetables, snap peas, and carved mushrooms. Stir-fry for around 5 mins 'til the vegetables are soft-crisp.
3. Inside your small container, whisk collectively low-sodium soy sauce, crushed garlic, grated ginger, and the cornstarch-water solution to form the sauce.
4. Pour your sauce over the vegetables then stir till the sauce denses.
5. Present your vegetable stir-fry over cooked brown rice.

Per serving: Calories: 230kcal; Fat: 3g; Carbs: 45g; Protein: 6g; Sodium: 390mg

56. *Baked Cod with Mediterranean Herbs*

Preparation time: 15 mins

Cooking time: 20 mins

Servings: 4

Ingredients:

- 4 cod fillets
- 2 tbsps fresh lemon juice
- 2 tbsps extra-virgin olive oil
- 2 pieces garlic, crushed
- 1 tsp dried oregano
- 1 tsp dried thyme
- 1/2 tsp paprika
- Salt and pepper as required
- Lemon wedges for garnish (elective)

Directions:

1. Warm up your oven to 375 deg.F.
2. In your little jar, mix together the fresh lemon juice, extra virgin olive oil, crushed garlic, paprika, dried thyme, dried oregano, and salt and pepper.
3. Put your cod fillets in your baking dish then spray the herb and lemon solution over them.
4. Bake for around 15-20 minsor 'til the cod flakes simply using a fork.
5. Garnish using lemon wedges if wanted.
6. Present hot.

Per serving: Calories: 180kcal; Fat: 7g; Carbs: 1g; Protein: 27g; Sodium: 180mg

57. *Turkey and Spinach Meatballs with Tomato Sauce*

Preparation time: 20 mins

Cooking time: 20 mins

Servings: 4

Ingredients:

- 1 lb. lean ground turkey
- 2 teacups fresh spinach leaves, severed
- 1/2 teacup whole wheat breadcrumbs
- 1/4 teacup grated Parmesan cheese
- 1 egg
- 2 pieces garlic, crushed
- 1/2 tsp dried basil
- 1/2 tsp dried oregano
- Salt and pepper as required
- 2 teacups low-sodium tomato sauce

Directions:

1. Inside your big container, blend lean ground turkey, severed fresh spinach, whole wheat breadcrumbs, grated Parmesan cheese, egg, crushed garlic, dried basil, dried oregano, salt, and pepper.
2. Mix till thoroughly blended.
3. Shape your solution into meatballs, around 1" in diameter.
4. In your skillet, heat a bit of olive oil in a middling temp.
5. Include the meatballs then cook for around 8-10 mins, mixing irregularly 'til browned on all sides.
6. Pour in low-sodium tomato sauce then simmer for an extra 10 mins 'til the meatballs are cooked through.
7. Present hot over whole wheat pasta or with a side of vegetables.

Per serving: Calories: 290kcal; Fat: 10g; Carbs: 21g; Protein: 27g; Sodium: 480mg

58. *Chickpea and Spinach Stew*

Preparation time: 15 mins

Cooking time: 25 mins

Servings: 4

Ingredients:

- 2 tins (15 oz. each) chickpeas, that is drained and washed
- 4 teacups fresh spinach leaves
- 1 onion, finely severed
- 2 pieces garlic, crushed
- 1 tin (14 oz.) cubed tomatoes
- 1 tsp ground cumin
- 1/2 tsp smoked paprika
- 1/4 tsp cayenne pepper (regulate as required)
- 2 tbsps olive oil
- Salt and pepper as required

Directions:

1. Inside your big griddle, warm olive oil in a middling temp.
2. Include finely severed onion then cook till translucent.
3. Stir in crushed garlic then cook for an extramin.
4. Include ground cumin, smoked paprika, and cayenne pepper. Cook for 1-2 mins 'til fragrant.
5. Pour in cubed tomatoes and chickpeas. Flavourusing salt and pepper.
6. Simmer for around 15 mins, mixing irregularly.
7. Stir in fresh spinach leaves then cook till wilted.
8. Present warm.

Per serving: Calories: 280kcal; Fat: 8g; Carbs: 45g; Protein: 13g; Sodium: 440mg

59. *Lemon Garlic Chicken with Asparagus*

Preparation time: 10 mins

Cooking time: 20 mins

Servings: 4

Ingredients:

- 4 boneless, skinless chicken breasts
- 1 bunch asparagus, clipped
- 4 pieces garlic, crushed
- Zest and juice of 1 lemon
- 2 tbsps fresh parsley, severed
- 2 tbsps olive oil
- Salt and pepper as required

Directions:

1. Flavour your chicken breasts using salt, pepper, and half of the crushed garlic.
2. Inside your big griddle, warm olive oil in a med-high temp.
3. Include the chicken breasts then cook for around 5-7 minson all side still they are cooked through and browned.
4. Take out your chicken from your griddle then put away.
5. Inside the similar griddle, include clipped asparagus and the remaining crushed garlic.
6. Cook for around 5 mins 'til the asparagus is soft-crisp.
7. Return the cooked chicken to your griddle.
8. Include lemon zest, lemon juice, and severed fresh parsley.
9. Cook for an extra 2-3 mins.
10. Present warm.

Per serving: Calories: 250kcal; Fat: 9g; Carbs: 6g; Protein: 36g; Sodium: 140mg

60. *Baked Eggplant Parmesan*

Preparation time: 20 mins

Cooking time: 30 mins

Servings: 4

Ingredients:

- 2 big eggplants, carved into rounds
- 2 teacups whole wheat breadcrumbs
- 1 teacup grated Parmesan cheese
- 2 teacups low-sodium marinara sauce
- 2 teacups shredded mozzarella cheese
- 2 tbsps olive oil
- Fresh basil leaves for garnish (elective)
- Salt and pepper as required

Directions:

1. Warm up your oven to 375 deg.F.
2. Put your eggplant rounds on your baking sheet, brush with olive oil, and flavourusing salt and pepper.
3. Bake for around 15-20 mins 'til the eggplant is soft and slightly browned.
4. In a shallow dish, blend whole wheat breadcrumbs and grated Parmesan cheese.
5. Drizzle some marinara sauce onto a different baking dish.
6. Dip each baked eggplant round into the breadcrumb solution, covering all sides, and put it in the baking dish with marinara sauce.
7. Repeat till you have a single layer of eggplant.
8. Top with shredded mozzarella cheese and repeat the layering process till all eggplant is used.
9. Bake for around 20-25 mins 'til the cheese is bubbly and golden.
10. Garnish using fresh basil leaves if wanted.
11. Present hot over whole wheat pasta.

Per serving: Calories: 450kcal; Fat: 17g; Carbs: 51g; Protein: 27g; Sodium: 680mg

61.Mushroom and Spinach Stuffed Portobello Mushrooms

Preparation time: 15 mins

Cooking time: 20 mins

Servings: 4

Ingredients:

- 4 large Portobello mushrooms, stems removed
- 2 teacups fresh spinach leaves, severed
- 1 teacup cubed mushrooms (use mushroom stems)
- 1/2 teacup cubed onion
- 2 pieces garlic, crushed
- 1/4 teacup shredded mozzarella cheese
- 2 tbsps olive oil
- 1/2 tsp dried thyme
- Salt and pepper as required

Directions:

1. Warm up your oven to 375 deg.F.
2. Inside your big griddle, warm olive oil in a middling temp.
3. Include cubed mushroom stems, cubed onion, and crushed garlic. Cook for around 5 mins 'til softened.
4. Stir in severed fresh spinach and dried thyme. Cook for an extra 2-3 mins 'til the spinach wilts.
5. Flavourusing salt and pepper.

6. Put your Portobello mushrooms on your baking sheet, gill side up.
7. Fill each mushroom cap using the spinach and mushroom solution.
8. Top with shredded mozzarella cheese.
9. Bake for around 15-20 mins 'til the mushrooms are soft then the cheese is dissolved and bubbly.
10. Present warm.

Per serving: Calories: 150kcal; Fat: 9g; Carbs: 12g; Protein: 8g; Sodium: 230mg

62. *Grilled Tofu with Peanut Sauce*

Preparation time: 15 mins

Cooking time: 10 mins

Servings: 4

Ingredients:

- 1 block extra-firm tofu, pressed and carved into planks
- 1/4 teacup low-sodium peanut butter
- 2 tbsps low-sodium soy sauce
- 2 tbsps fresh lime juice
- 1 tbsp honey
- 2 pieces garlic, crushed
- 1 tsp fresh ginger, grated
- 2 tbsps water
- Severed cilantro and crushed peanuts for garnish (elective)

Directions:

1. Warm up your grill to med-high temp.
2. Inside your container, whisk collectively low-sodium peanut butter, low-sodium soy sauce, fresh lime juice, honey, crushed garlic, grated ginger, and water to form the peanut sauce.
3. Grill tofu planks for around 4-5 minson all side still grill marks appear then the tofu is heated through.
4. Brush each tofu plank with peanut sauce while grilling.
5. Present grilled tofu with extra peanut sauce on the side.
6. Garnish using severed cilantro and crushed peanuts if wanted.
7. Present warm.

Per serving: Calories: 220kcal; Fat: 13g; Carbs: 13g; Protein: 16g; Sodium: 250mg

63. *Spinach and Feta Stuffed Pork Tenderloin*

Preparation time: 20 mins

Cooking time: 35 mins

Servings: 4

Ingredients:

- 1 pork tenderloin (about 1 lb.)
- 2 teacups fresh spinach leaves
- 1/2 teacup smashed feta cheese
- 2 pieces garlic, crushed
- 1 tsp dried oregano
- Salt and pepper as required
- Olive oil for cooking

Directions:

1. Warm up your oven to 375 deg.F.
2. Butterfly the pork tenderloin by slicing it lengthwise without cutting all the way through. Open it like a book.
3. Flavour your inside with salt, pepper, and dried oregano.
4. Layer fresh spinach leaves, smashed feta cheese, and crushed garlic over the pork.
5. Using kitchen twine, secure the pork tenderloin as it rolls up.
6. In your large ovenproof skillet, warm olive oil inside a med-high temp.
7. Sear until browned on all sides of the pork tenderloin.
8. Bring your skillet to your warmed up oven and roast for around 20-25 minsor 'til your pork reaches an inside temperature of 145 deg.F.
9. Take out from the oven and allow it to relax for a few minsprior to cutting.
10. Present warm.

Per serving: Calories: 220kcal; Fat: 9g; Carbs: 1g; Protein: 32g; Sodium: 380mg

64. *Mediterranean Couscous Salad*

Preparation time: 15 mins

Cooking time: 5 mins

Servings: 4

Ingredients:

- 1 teacup whole wheat couscous, cooked and cooled
- 1 teacup cucumber, cubed
- 1 teacup cherry tomatoes, divided
- 1/2 teacup Kalamata olives, that is eroded and carved
- 1/2 teacup smashed feta cheese
- 1/4 teacup red onion, finely severed
- 2 tbsps extra-virgin olive oil

- 2 tbsps fresh lemon juice
- 2 tbsps fresh parsley, severed
- Salt and pepper as required

Directions:

1. Inside your big container, blend cooked and cooled whole wheat couscous, cubed cucumber, divided cherry tomatoes, carved Kalamata olives, smashed feta cheese, and finely severed red onion.
2. Inside your small container, whisk collectively extra-virgin olive oil, fresh lemon juice, severed fresh parsley, salt, and pepper to form your dressing.
3. Pour the dressing over the salad, then give it a light shake to distribute it evenly.
4. Present chilled.

Per serving: Calories: 270kcal; Fat: 12g; Carbs: 34g; Protein: 9g; Sodium: 470mg

65. *Roasted Vegetable and Chickpea Bowl*

Preparation time: 15 mins

Cooking time: 30 mins

Servings: 4

Ingredients:

- 2 teacups mixed vegetables (e.g., bell peppers, cherry tomatoes, and zucchini), cubed
- 1 tin (15 oz.) chickpeas, that is drained and washed
- 1 teacup cooked quinoa
- 2 tbsps extra-virgin olive oil
- 1 tsp dried oregano
- 1/2 tsp smoked paprika
- Salt and pepper as required
- 1/4 teacup fresh basil leaves, severed
- 2 tbsps balsamic vinegar

Directions:

1. Warm up your oven to 400 deg.F.
2. Inside your big container, toss cubed mixed vegetables and chickpeas with extra-virgin olive oil, dried oregano, smoked paprika, salt, and pepper.
3. Disperse the solution on your baking sheet.
4. Roast in the oven for around 25-30 mins 'til the vegetables are soft and slightly caramelized.
5. Inside your container, blend cooked quinoa, roasted vegetables, chickpeas, severed fresh basil, and balsamic vinegar.
6. Shake to blend.
7. Present warm or at room temp.

Per serving: Calories: 310kcal; Fat: 10g; Carbs: 47g; Protein: 10g; Sodium: 340mg

66. Quinoa and Black Bean Stuffed Acorn Squash

Preparation time: 15 mins

Cooking time: 45 mins

Servings: 4

Ingredients:

- 2 acorn squashes, divided and seeds removed
- 1 teacup quinoa, that is washed then cooked
- 1 tin (15 oz.) black beans, that is drained and washed
- 1 teacup cubed tomatoes (canned or fresh)
- 1/2 teacup cubed red onion
- 2 pieces garlic, crushed
- 1 tsp ground cumin
- 1/2 tsp chili powder
- Salt and pepper as required
- Fresh cilantro leaves for garnish (elective)

Directions:

1. Warm up your oven to 375 deg.F.
2. Place the halves of the acorn squash, cut side down, onto the baking sheet.
3. Bake for around 30-35 mins 'til the squash is soft.
4. While squash is baking, prepare the filling. Inside your big container, blend cooked quinoa, black beans, cubed tomatoes, cubed red onion, crushed garlic, ground cumin, chili powder, salt, and pepper.
5. Once the squash is cooked, flip the halves over and stuff each with the quinoa and black bean solution.
6. Return to the oven then bake for an extra 10-15 mins.
7. Garnish using fresh cilantro leaves if wanted.
8. Present hot.

Per serving: Calories: 330kcal; Fat: 2g; Carbs: 65g; Protein: 12g; Sodium: 310mg

67. Spaghetti Aglio e Olio with Spinach

Preparation time: 10 mins

Cooking time: 15 mins

Servings: 4

Ingredients:

- 8 oz. whole wheat spaghetti
- 4 pieces garlic, thinly carved
- 1/4 teacup extra-virgin olive oil
- 1/4 tsp red pepper flakes
- 4 teacups fresh spinach leaves

- Zest and juice of 1 lemon
- Salt and pepper as required
- Grated Parmesan cheese for garnish (elective)

Directions:

1. Cook whole wheat spaghetti using package guide line still al dente. Drain and put away.
2. Inside your big griddle, warm extra-virgin olive oil in a middling temp.
3. Add the red pepper flakes and finely sliced garlic. Cook for around 2-3 mins 'til the garlic is fragrant and mildly golden.
4. Stir in fresh spinach leaves then cook for an extra 2-3 mins 'til wilted.
5. Include cooked spaghetti to your griddle, along with lemon zest and lemon juice.
6. Shake to blend and flavourusing salt and pepper.
7. Garnish using grated Parmesan cheese if wanted.
8. Present hot.

Per serving: Calories: 280kcal; Fat: 13g; Carbs: 35g; Protein: 8g; Sodium: 190mg

68. *Grilled Turkey Burger with Avocado*

Preparation time: 15 mins

Cooking time: 10 mins

Servings: 4

Ingredients:

- 1 lb. lean ground turkey
- 1/2 teacup rolled oats (for binding)
- 1/4 teacup finely severed red onion
- 1/4 teacup severed fresh cilantro
- 1 tsp ground cumin
- 1/2 tsp chili powder
- Salt and pepper as required
- 4 whole wheat burger buns
- 1 ripe avocado, carved
- Lettuce, tomato slices, and low-fat yogurt (for toppings)

Directions:

1. Inside your container, blend lean ground turkey, rolled oats, severed red onion, severed fresh cilantro, ground cumin, chili powder, salt, and pepper.
2. Shape your solution into four burger patties.
3. Warm up your grill to med-high temp.
4. Grill the turkey burgers for around 4-5 minson all side still they are cooked through and have grill marks.
5. For a minute or two, toast the whole wheat burger buns on the grill.

6. Assemble the burgers with lettuce, tomato slices, carved avocado, and a dollop of low-fat yogurt.
7. Present warm.

Per serving: Calories: 350kcal; Fat: 13g; Carbs: 30g; Protein: 28g; Sodium: 400mg

69. *Lemon Herb Quinoa with Grilled Chicken*

Preparation time: 15 mins

Cooking time: 20 mins

Servings: 4

Ingredients:

- 1 teacup quinoa, that is washed then cooked
- 4 boneless, skinless chicken breasts
- Zest and juice of 1 lemon
- 2 tbsps fresh parsley, severed
- 2 tbsps fresh basil, severed
- 1 tbsp extra-virgin olive oil
- Salt and pepper as required

Directions:

1. Flavour your chicken breasts with salt, pepper, lemon zest, and severed fresh basil.
2. Warm up your grill to med-high temp.
3. Grill the chicken breasts for around 6-7 minson all side still they are cooked through and have grill marks.
4. Inside your container, blend cooked quinoa, lemon juice, severed fresh parsley, extra-virgin olive oil, salt, and pepper.
5. Present your grilled chicken on a bed of lemon herb quinoa.
6. Garnish using additional fresh herbs if wanted.
7. Present warm.

Per serving: Calories: 340kcal; Fat: 7g; Carbs: 35g; Protein: 34g; Sodium: 110mg

70. *Baked Zucchini Boats with Ground Turkey*

Preparation time: 20 mins

Cooking time: 30 mins

Servings: 4

Ingredients:

- 4 medium zucchinis
- 1 lb. lean ground turkey
- 1 teacup cubed tomatoes (canned or fresh)
- 1/2 teacup cubed onion
- 2 pieces garlic, crushed

- 1 tsp dried oregano
- 1/2 tsp dried basil
- Salt and pepper as required
- 1/4 teacup shredded low-fat mozzarella cheese
- Severed fresh basil leaves for garnish (elective)

Directions:
1. Warm up your oven to 375 deg.F.
2. Slice the zucchinis lengthwise in half, then remove the meat, leaving about 1/4 of an inch of the zucchini shell intact.
3. In your skillet, cook lean ground turkey in a med-high temp till browned.
4. Include cubed tomatoes, cubed onion, crushed garlic, dried oregano, dried basil, salt, and pepper to your griddle. Cook for 5 mins.
5. Fill the zucchini boats with the turkey solution.
6. Put your filled zucchini boats in your baking dish.
7. Cover using foil then bake for around 20-25 mins 'til the zucchinis are soft.
8. Take out foil, spray shredded low-fat mozzarella cheese on top, then bake for an extra 5 mins 'til the cheese is dissolved and bubbly.
9. Garnish using severed fresh basil leaves if wanted.
10. Present warm.

Per serving: Calories: 240kcal; Fat: 8g; Carbs: 16g; Protein: 26g; Sodium: 220mg

71. Spinach and Mushroom Risotto
Preparation time: 10 mins
Cooking time: 30 mins
Servings: 4
Ingredients:
- 1 teacup Arborio rice
- 8 oz. fresh mushrooms, carved
- 4 teacups low-sodium vegetable broth
- 2 teacups fresh spinach leaves
- 1/2 teacup cubed onion
- 2 pieces garlic, crushed
- 1/4 teacup grated Parmesan cheese
- 2 tbsps olive oil
- Salt and pepper as required

Directions:
1. Inside a saucepot, heat the low-sodium vegetable broth over low heat. Keep it warm.
2. Inside your big griddle, warm olive oil in a middling temp.
3. Include cubed onion then cook till translucent.

4. Stir in crushed garlic and carved mushrooms. Cook for around 5 mins 'til the mushrooms are browned.

5. Include Arborio rice then cook for 2-3 mins, stirring constantly.

6. Start giving the heated vegetable broth one scoop at a moment while swirling the mixture constantly till the majority of the liquid has been soaked prior to including more of it.

7. Last this process till the rice is creamy and soft, which should take about 20-25 mins.

8. Stir in fresh spinach leaves till they wilt.

9. Remove from the fire and add the grated Parmesan cheese.

10. Flavourusing salt and pepper as required.

11. Present hot.

Per serving: Calories: 290kcal; Fat: 8g; Carbs: 46g; Protein: 8g; Sodium: 240mg

72. *Honey Mustard Glazed Salmon*

Preparation time: 10 mins

Cooking time: 15 mins

Servings: 4

Ingredients:

- 4 salmon fillets
- 1/4 teacup Dijon mustard
- 2 tbsps honey
- 1 tbsp fresh lemon juice
- 1 piece garlic, crushed
- 1/2 tsp dried dill
- Salt and pepper as required
- Lemon wedges & fresh dill sprigs for garnish (elective)

Directions:

1. Warm up your oven to 375 deg.F.

2. Inside your container, whisk collectively Dijon mustard, honey, fresh lemon juice, crushed garlic, dried dill, salt, and pepper to form the honey mustard glaze.

3. Put the salmon fillets on the parchment paper-lined baking sheet.

4. With some reserved for later, brush the salmon fillets with the honey mustard glaze.

5. Bake for around 12-15 mins 'til the salmon flakes easily using a fork.

6. Spray the remaining honey mustard glaze over the cooked salmon.

7. Garnish using lemon wedges and fresh dill sprigs if wanted.

8. Present hot.

Per serving: Calories: 300kcal; Fat: 12g; Carbs: 12g; Protein: 33g; Sodium: 320mg

Snacks and Desserts: Healthy Nibbles and Sweet Treats

73.   *Sliced Apple with Almond Butter*

Preparation time: 5 mins

Cooking time: None

Servings: 1

Ingredients:

- 1 medium apple, carved
- 2 tbsps almond butter

Directions:

1. Slice the apple into thin wedges.
2. Dip the apple slices in almond butter.
3. Enjoy this delicious and healthy snack!

Per serving: Calories: 250kcal; Fat: 15g; Carbs: 30g; Protein: 5g; Sodium: 0mg

74.   *Carrot Sticks with Hummus*

Preparation time: 10 mins

Cooking time: None

Servings: 2

Ingredients:

- 4 medium carrots, cut into sticks
- 1/2 teacup hummus

Directions:

1. Wash and peel the carrots, then cut them into sticks.
2. Present your carrot sticks with a side of hummus for dipping.
3. Enjoy this crunchy and satisfying snack!

Per serving: Calories: 120kcal; Fat: 6g; Carbs: 14g; Protein: 4g; Sodium: 180mg

75.   *Trail Mix with Nuts and Dried Fruit*

Preparation time: 5 mins

Cooking time: None

Servings: 2

Ingredients:

- 1/2 teacup mixed nuts (almonds, cashews, walnuts)
- 1/4 teacup dried cranberries
- 1/4 teacup raisins

Directions:

1. Combine the mixed nuts, dried cranberries, and raisins in a bowl.
2. Mix well to create your own healthy trail mix.

3. Portion into individual servings for a quick and nutritious snack!

Per serving: Calories: 250kcal; Fat: 18g; Carbs: 22g; Protein: 5g; Sodium: 5mg

76. *Mixed Berries with a Spray of Cinnamon*

Preparation time: 5 mins

Cooking time: None

Servings: 1

Ingredients:

- 1 teacup mixed berries (strawberries, blueberries, raspberries)
- A spray of ground cinnamon

Directions:

1. Wash the mixed berries and place them inside a container.
2. Spray a tweak of ground cinnamon over the berries.
3. Gently toss to blend and savor the natural sweetness of the berries.

Per serving: Calories: 80kcal; Fat: 0g; Carbs: 20g; Protein: 1g; Sodium: 0mg

77. *Dark Chocolate Covered Almonds*

Preparation time: 10 mins

Cooking time: None

Servings: 2

Ingredients:

- 1/2 teacup dark chocolate chips (cocoa 70%)
- 1/2 teacup whole almonds

Directions:

1. Melt your dark chocolate chips in a microwave-safe bowl in 30-second intervals, stirring till smooth.
2. After dipping each almond into the melted chocolate, place them on a pan lined with parchment paper.
3. Allow the chocolate to cool and harden.
4. Enjoy these delightful chocolate-covered almonds as a satisfying snack!

Per serving: Calories: 200kcal; Fat: 15g; Carbs: 15g; Protein: 4g; Sodium: 0mg

78. *Baked Sweet Potato Fries*

Preparation time: 10 mins

Cooking time: 25 mins

Servings: 2

Ingredients:

- 2 medium sweet potatoes, cut into fries

- 1 tbsp olive oil
- 1/2 tsp paprika
- 1/2 tsp garlic powder
- Salt and pepper as required

Directions:

1. Warm up your oven to 425 deg.F.
2. Inside your container, toss sweet potato fries with paprika, olive oil, salt, garlic powder, and pepper.
3. Disperse your fries in a single layer on your baking sheet.
4. Bake 20-25 mins, flipping them halfway through, 'til they are crispy and mildly browned.
5. Present as a nutritious alternative to traditional fries!

Per serving: Calories: 180kcal; Fat: 6g; Carbs: 30g; Protein: 3g; Sodium: 90mg

79. *Cottage Cheese with Pineapple*

Preparation time: 5 mins

Cooking time: None

Servings: 2

Ingredients:

- 1 teacup low-fat cottage cheese
- 1 teacup cubed pineapple (fresh or canned in juice, drained)

Directions:

1. Split your cottage cheese into two containers.
2. Top each bowl with half of the cubed pineapple.
3. Enjoy this simple and protein-packed snack or light meal!

Per serving: Calories: 180kcal; Fat: 2g; Carbs: 26g; Protein: 15g; Sodium: 400mg

80. *Banana Slices with Peanut Butter*

Preparation time: 5 mins

Cooking time: None

Servings: 2

Ingredients:

- 2 medium bananas, carved
- 4 tbsps natural peanut butter

Directions:

1. Slice the bananas into rounds.
2. Disperse 2 tbsps of your peanut butter on each serving plate.
3. Dip banana slices into the peanut butter and relish this tasty and filling snack!

Per serving: Calories: 250kcal; Fat: 14g; Carbs: 30g; Protein: 6g; Sodium: 100mg

81. *Frozen Yogurt with Fresh Strawberries*
Preparation time: 5 mins
Cooking time: None
Servings: 2
Ingredients:

- 1 teacup low-fat vanilla frozen yogurt
- 1 teacup fresh strawberries, carved

Directions:

1. Scoop the frozen yogurt into two containers.
2. Top each bowl with carved strawberries.
3. Savor the combination of creamy yogurt and sweet strawberries for a refreshing dessert or snack!

Per serving: Calories: 150kcal; Fat: 2g; Carbs: 30g; Protein: 4g; Sodium: 70mg

82. *Cucumber Slices with Tzatziki*
Preparation time: 10 mins
Cooking time: None
Servings: 2
Ingredients:

- 1 cucumber, thinly carved
- 1/2 teacup tzatziki sauce (low-fat, if available)

Directions:

1. Arrange the cucumber slices on a plate.
2. Present with tzatziki sauce for dipping.
3. Enjoy this refreshing and low-calorie snack!

Per serving: Calories: 60kcal; Fat: 3g; Carbs: 8g; Protein: 2g; Sodium: 75mg

83. *Air-Popped Popcorn with Herbs*
Preparation time: 5 mins
Cooking time: 5 mins
Servings: 2
Ingredients:

- 1/2 teacup popcorn kernels
- 1 tbsp olive oil
- 1 tsp dried herbs (e.g., as oregano, thyme, or rosemary)
- Salt and pepper as required

Directions:

1. Air-pop the popcorn according to the manufacturer's instructions.

2. Spray olive oil over the popped popcorn.
3. Spray dried herbs, salt, and pepper over the popcorn.
4. Shake to cover evenly and relish this flavorful and low-sodium snack!

Per serving: Calories: 100kcal; Fat: 4g; Carbs: 14g; Protein: 2g; Sodium: 0mg

84. *Berry Smoothie with Spinach*

Preparation time: 5 mins

Cooking time: None

Servings: 1

Ingredients:

- 1 teacup mixed berries (strawberries, blueberries, raspberries)
- 1 teacup fresh spinach leaves
- 1/2 teacup low-fat yogurt
- 1/2 teacup water
- 1 tsp honey (elective)

Directions:

1. Place mixed berries, fresh spinach, yogurt, water, and honey (if wanted) inside a mixer.
2. Blend till smooth and creamy.
3. Pour into a glass and relish this nutrient-packed smoothie!

Per serving: Calories: 150kcal; Fat: 2g; Carbs: 28g; Protein: 7g; Sodium: 100mg

85. *Rice Cakes with Avocado*

Preparation time: 5 mins

Cooking time: None

Servings: 2

Ingredients:

- 2 rice cakes (choose low-sodium options)
- 1 ripe avocado
- Salt and pepper as required
- A spray of paprika (elective)

Directions:

1. Cut your avocado in 1/2, take out the pit, then scoop out the flesh into your container.
2. Mash the avocado using a fork and flavourusing salt and pepper.
3. Disperse the mashed avocado evenly onto the rice cakes.
4. Spray using paprika if wanted and relish this simple and healthy snack!

Per serving: Calories: 150kcal; Fat: 10g; Carbs: 14g; Protein: 2g; Sodium: 0mg

86. *Roasted Chickpeas with Herbs*

Preparation time: 10 mins

Cooking time: 30 mins

Servings: 4

Ingredients:

- 2 tins (15 oz. each) chickpeas, that is drained and washed
- 2 tbsps olive oil
- 1 tsp dried herbs (e.g., as thyme or rosemary)
- Salt and pepper as required

Directions:

1. Warm up your oven to 400 deg.F.
2. Pat your chickpeas dry using a paper towel and put them on your baking sheet.
3. Once the chickpeas have been sprayed with olive oil, season with salt, pepper, and dry herbs.
4. Shake to cover evenly, then roast in the oven for around 30 minsor 'til they become crispy.
5. Allowing them to cool will allow you to enjoy this crispy, high-protein snack!

Per serving: Calories: 200kcal; Fat: 7g; Carbs: 28g; Protein: 7g; Sodium: 300mg

87. *Sliced Cucumber with Olive Oil and Vinegar*

Preparation time: 5 mins

Cooking time: None

Servings: 2

Ingredients:

- 1 cucumber, thinly carved
- 1 tbsp extra-virgin olive oil
- 1 tbsp vinegar (balsamic, red wine, or white wine)
- Salt and pepper as required
- Fresh herbs (elective, for garnish)

Directions:

1. Arrange the cucumber slices on a plate.
2. Spray olive oil and vinegar over the cucumber slices.
3. Flavourusing salt and pepper.
4. Garnish using fresh herbs if wanted.
5. Enjoy this refreshing and low-calorie snack!

Per serving: Calories: 70kcal; Fat: 7g; Carbs: 2g; Protein: 0g; Sodium: 5mg

88. *Chia Seed Pudding with Berries*

Preparation time: 10 mins (plus chilling time)

Cooking time: None

Servings: 2

Ingredients:

- 1/4 teacup chia seeds
- 1 teacup unsweetened almond milk
- 1/2 tsp vanilla extract
- 1 teacup mixed berries (strawberries, blueberries, raspberries)
- Honey or maple syrup (elective, for sweetness)

Directions:

1. Inside your container, blend chia seeds, almond milk, and vanilla extract.
2. Stir well, cover, then put in the fridge for almost 2 hrs or overnight, allowing it to thicken.
3. Prior to presenting, layer the chia pudding with mixed berries.
4. Sweeten using honey or maple syrup if wanted.
5. Enjoy this nutritious and fiber-rich dessert or breakfast!

Per serving: Calories: 160kcal; Fat: 9g; Carbs: 16g; Protein: 4g; Sodium: 90mg

89. *Baked Apple with Cinnamon and Walnuts*

Preparation time: 10 mins

Cooking time: 20 mins

Servings: 2

Ingredients:

- 2 apples
- 1/4 teacup severed walnuts
- 1 tsp ground cinnamon
- 1 tbsp honey (elective)

Directions:

1. Warm up your oven to 350 deg.F.
2. Core your apples and take out the seeds, leaving the bottom intact.
3. Inside your small container, mix severed walnuts and cinnamon.
4. Stuff each apple with the walnut-cinnamon solution.
5. Spray using honey if wanted.
6. Bake for about 20 minutes, or until the apples are tender.
7. Enjoy Savor this comforting and warm dessert!

Per serving: Calories: 200kcal; Fat: 9g; Carbs: 32g; Protein: 2g; Sodium: 0mg

90. *Almond and Date Energy Bites*

Preparation time: 15 mins

Cooking time: None

Servings: 12 bites

Ingredients:

- 1 teacup eroded dates
- 1 teacup almonds
- 2 tbsps chia seeds
- 1/2 tsp vanilla extract
- Tweak of salt

Directions:

1. Place dates, almonds, chia seeds, vanilla extract, and a tweak of salt in blending container.
2. Pulse until the mixture resembles sticky dough.
3. Create little, bite-sized balls out of the dough.
4. Store in the refrigerator and relish these energy-boosting bites whenever you need a snack!

Per serving: Calories: 90kcal; Fat: 4g; Carbs: 13g; Protein: 2g; Sodium: 0mg

91. *Greek Yogurt Bark with Fruit*

Preparation time: 10 mins (plus freezing time)

Cooking time: None

Servings: 4

Ingredients:

- 2 teacups Greek yogurt (low-fat or non-fat)
- 1 teacup mixed fruit (strawberries, blueberries, kiwi, etc.), severed
- 2 tbsps honey
- 1/4 teacup granola (elective)

Directions:

1. Cover a baking sheet with parchment paper.
2. Disperse Greek yogurt evenly on the parchment paper.
3. Spray severed fruit over the yogurt.
4. Spray using honey.
5. If desired, spray granola on top for added crunch.
6. Freeze for almost 2 hrsor 'til firm.
7. Break into pieces and relish this cool and protein-rich treat!

Per serving: Calories: 140kcal; Fat: 0g; Carbs: 26g; Protein: 9g; Sodium: 30mg

92. *Spinach and Feta Mini Quiches*

Preparation time: 15 mins

Cooking time: 20 mins

Servings: 6 mini quiches

Ingredients:

- 4 large eggs
- 1/4 teacup milk (low-fat or plant-based)
- 1 teacup fresh spinach, severed
- 1/4 teacup smashed feta cheese
- Salt and pepper as required

Directions:

1. Warm up oven to 375 deg. F then oil a muffin tin.
2. Inside your container, whisk collectively the eggs and milk.
3. Flavourusing salt and pepper.
4. Split your severed spinach and feta cheese evenly among the muffin tin teacups.
5. Pour your egg solution over the spinach and feta.
6. Bake for around 20 minsor 'til the quiches are set and mildly browned.
7. Let them to cool slightly before serving these protein-packed mini quiches!

Per serving: Calories: 90kcal; Fat: 6g; Carbs: 2g; Protein: 6g; Sodium: 120mg

93. *Whole Wheat Banana Bread*

Preparation time: 15 mins

Cooking time: 50-60 mins

Servings: 10 slices

Ingredients:

- 2 ripe bananas, mashed
- 1/4 teacup olive oil
- 1/4 teacup honey or maple syrup
- 2 large eggs
- 1 tsp vanilla extract
- 1 1/2 teacups whole wheat flour
- 1 tsp baking soda
- 1/2 tsp salt
- 1/2 tsp ground cinnamon

Directions:

1. Warm up your oven to 350 deg.F. Grease and flour a loaf pan.
2. Inside your container, mix mashed bananas, olive oil, honey or maple syrup, eggs, and vanilla extract.

3. Inside your additional container, whisk collectively whole wheat flour, baking soda, salt, and cinnamon.
4. Mix your wet & dry component still just incorporated.
5. Pour batter into your arranged loaf pan.
6. Bake 50-60 minsor 'til a toothpick immersed into the center comes out clean.
7. Let your banana bread cool prior to cutting and enjoying this wholesome treat!

Per serving: Calories: 160kcal; Fat: 6g; Carbs: 26g; Protein: 3g; Sodium: 210mg

94. *Oatmeal Cookies with Raisins*

Preparation time: 15 mins
Cooking time: 10-12 mins
Servings: About 24 cookies
Ingredients:

- 1 teacup old-fashioned oats
- 1/2 teacup whole wheat flour
- 1/2 teacup unsweetened applesauce
- 1/4 teacup honey or maple syrup
- 1/4 teacup raisins
- 1/2 tsp ground cinnamon
- 1/4 tsp baking soda
- 1/4 tsp salt

Directions:

1. Warm up your oven to 350 deg. F then line your baking sheet using parchment paper.
2. Combine oats, whole wheat flour, ground cinnamon, baking soda, and salt in your container.
3. Inside your distinct container, mix applesauce, honey or maple syrup, and raisins.
4. Mix the wet & dry component still a cookie dough forms.
5. Spoon dough onto the baking sheet that has been prepared.
6. Use the back of a fork to flatten each biscuit.
7. Bake for 10-12 minsor 'til the edges are golden brown.
8. Allow your cookies to cool before enjoying these fiber-rich treats!

Per serving: Calories: 50kcal; Fat: 0.5g; Carbs: 11g; Protein: 1g; Sodium: 40mg

95. *Avocado Chocolate Mousse*

Preparation time: 10 mins

Cooking time: None

Servings: 2

Ingredients:

- 1 ripe avocado
- 2 tbsps unsweetened cocoa powder
- 2 tbsps honey or maple syrup
- 1/2 tsp vanilla extract
- A tweak of salt

Directions:

1. Scoop the flesh of the ripe avocado into a blender or blending container.
2. Include cocoa powder, honey or maple syrup, vanilla extract, and a tweak of salt.
3. Blend till smooth and creamy.
4. Split into serving teacups then put in the fridge for almost 30 mins before enjoying this guilt-free chocolate mousse!

Per serving: Calories: 200kcal; Fat: 11g; Carbs: 27g; Protein: 2g; Sodium: 10mg

96. *Frozen Banana Popsicles*

Preparation time: 10 mins (plus freezing time)

Cooking time: None

Servings: 4 popsicles

Ingredients:

- 2 ripe bananas
- 1/4 teacup plain Greek yogurt
- 1 tbsp honey or maple syrup
- 1/4 teacup severed nuts or granola (elective)

Directions:

1. Peel and cut the bananas in half.
2. Slide your popsicle stick into each side of a banana.
3. Inside your container, mix Greek yogurt and honey or maple syrup.
4. Dip each banana pop into the yogurt solution, allowing excess to drip off.
5. If desired, roll in severed nuts or granola for added texture.
6. Place on a tray lined using parchment paper and freeze for almost 2 hrsor 'til firm.
7. Enjoy these creamy and naturally sweet frozen popsicles!

Per serving: Calories: 90kcal; Fat: 1.5g; Carbs: 20g; Protein: 2g; Sodium: 0mg

Beverages: Hydration with a Purpose

97. *Infused Water with Lemon and Mint*

Preparation time: 5 mins

Cooking time: 0 mins

Servings: 1

Ingredients:

- 1 lemon, carved
- 5-6 fresh mint leaves
- 1 glass of water

Directions:

1. Fill a glass with water.
2. Include lemon slices and mint leaves.
3. Let it infuse for a refreshing, low-sodium drink.

Per serving: Calories: 0kcal; Fat: 0 g; Carbs: 0 g; Protein: 0 g; Sodium: 0mg

98. *Green Tea with a Slice of Orange*

Preparation time: 2 mins

Cooking time: 5 mins (for steeping)

Servings: 1

Ingredients:

- 1 green tea bag
- 1 slice of orange

Directions:

1. Put your green tea bag in a teacup.
2. Boil water then pour it over your tea bag.
3. Let it steep for 5 mins.
4. Include a slice of orange for flavor.

Per serving: Calories: 0kcal; Fat: 0 g; Carbs: 0 g; Protein: 0 g; Sodium: 0mg

99. *Freshly Squeezed Orange Juice*

Preparation time: 5 mins

Cooking time: 0 mins

Servings: 1

Ingredients:

- 2-3 fresh oranges

Directions:

1. Wash and peel the oranges.
2. Squeeze the juice using a manual juicer or by hand.

Per serving: Calories: 80kcal; Fat: 0 g; Carbs: 20 g; Protein: 1 g; Sodium: 0mg

100. *Cucumber and Lemon Water*

Preparation time: 5 mins

Cooking time: 0 mins

Servings: 1

Ingredients:

- 1/2 cucumber, carved
- 1 lemon, carved
- 1 glass of water

Directions:

1. Fill a glass with water.
2. Include cucumber and lemon slices.
3. Stir and relish this refreshing low-sodium drink.

Per serving: Calories: 10kcal; Fat: 0 g; Carbs: 3 g; Protein: 0 g; Sodium: 0mg

101. *Berry and Spinach Smoothie*

Preparation time: 5 mins

Cooking time: 0 mins

Servings: 1

Ingredients:

- 1 teacup fresh spinach leaves
- 1/2 teacup mixed berries (e.g., strawberries, blueberries, raspberries)
- 1/2 banana
- 1 tbsp olive oil

Directions:

1. Place spinach, mixed berries, banana, and olive oil inside a mixer.
2. Blend till smooth.

Per serving: Calories: 150kcal; Fat: 9 g; Carbs: 18 g; Protein: 2 g; Sodium: 10mg

102. *Iced Herbal Tea with Fresh Herbs*

Preparation time: 10 mins

Cooking time: 5 mins (for steeping)

Servings: 1

Ingredients:

- 1 herbal tea bag (e.g., chamomile, mint)
- Fresh herbs (e.g., mint, basil)
- Ice cubes

Directions:

1. Boil water and steep the herbal tea bag for 5 mins.
2. Let it cool and include fresh herbs for flavor.
3. Present over ice.

Per serving: Calories: 0kcal; Fat: 0 g; Carbs: 0 g; Protein: 0 g; Sodium: 0mg

103. *Coconut Water with a Splash of Lime*

Preparation time: 2 mins

Cooking time: 0 mins

Servings: 1

Ingredients:

- 1 teacup coconut water
- Juice of half a lime

Directions:

1. Combine coconut water and lime juice in a glass.
2. Stir well and present chilled.

Per serving: Calories: 46kcal; Fat: 0 g; Carbs: 11 g; Protein: 0 g; Sodium: 252mg

104. *Homemade Fruit Smoothie with Greek Yogurt*

Preparation time: 5 mins

Cooking time: 0 mins

Servings: 1

Ingredients:

- 1/2 teacup mixed berries (e.g., strawberries, blueberries, raspberries)
- 1/2 banana
- 1/2 teacup low-fat Greek yogurt
- 1 tbsp olive oil

Directions:

1. Place mixed berries, banana, Greek yogurt, and olive oil inside a mixer.
2. Blend till smooth.

Per serving: Calories: 220kcal; Fat: 10 g; Carbs: 27 g; Protein: 9 g; Sodium: 60mg

105. *Freshly Squeezed Grapefruit Juice*

Preparation time: 5 mins

Cooking time: 0 mins

Servings: 1

Ingredients:

- 1 fresh grapefruit

Directions:

1. Cut the grapefruit in half and juice it using a juicer or by hand.

Per serving: Calories: 52kcal; Fat: 0 g; Carbs: 13 g; Protein: 1 g; Sodium: 0mg

106. *Almond Milk with a Hint of Vanilla*

Preparation time: 5 mins

Cooking time: 0 mins

Servings: 1

Ingredients:

- 1 teacup unsweetened almond milk
- 1/2 tsp pure vanilla extract

Directions:

1. Inside your glass, blend almond milk and vanilla extract.
2. Stir well and relish.

Per serving: Calories: 15kcal; Fat: 1 g; Carbs: 1 g; Protein: 0 g; Sodium: 150mg

107. *Sparkling Water with Lime Wedges*

Preparation time: 2 mins

Cooking time: 0 mins

Servings: 1

Ingredients:

- 1 teacup sparkling water
- Lime wedges for garnish

Directions:

1. Pour sparkling water into a glass.
2. Garnish using lime wedges.

Per serving: Calories: 0kcal; Fat: 0 g; Carbs: 0 g; Protein: 0 g; Sodium: 0mg

108. Spinach and Pineapple Smoothie

Preparation time: 5 mins

Cooking time: 0 mins

Servings: 1

Ingredients:

- 1 teacup fresh spinach leaves
- 1/2 teacup pineapple chunks
- 1/2 banana
- 1/2 teacup unsweetened almond milk

Directions:

1. Put spinach, pineapple chunks, banana, and almond milk inside a mixer.
2. Blend till smooth.

Per serving: Calories: 110kcal; Fat: 2 g; Carbs: 24 g; Protein: 2 g; Sodium: 80mg

109. Carrot and Ginger Juice

Preparation time: 5 mins

Cooking time: 0 mins

Servings: 1

Ingredients:

- 2 large carrots
- 1 small piece of fresh ginger

Directions:

1. Wash and peel the carrots.
2. Peel and chop the ginger.
3. Run the carrots and ginger through a juicer.

Per serving: Calories: 80kcal; Fat: 0 g; Carbs: 19 g; Protein: 2 g; Sodium: 80mg

110. *Berry Infused Iced Tea*

Preparation time: 10 mins

Cooking time: 5 mins (for steeping)

Servings: 1

Ingredients:

- 1 black tea bag
- 1/2 teacup mixed berries (e.g., strawberries, blueberries, raspberries)
- Ice cubes

Directions:

1. Boil water and steep the black tea bag for 5 mins.
2. Let it cool, then include mixed berries.
3. Present over ice.

Per serving: Calories: 10kcal; Fat: 0 g; Carbs: 3 g; Protein: 0 g; Sodium: 0mg

111. *Avocado and Banana Smoothie*

Preparation time: 5 mins

Cooking time: 0 mins

Servings: 1

Ingredients:

- 1/2 ripe avocado
- 1 ripe banana
- 1 teacup unsweetened almond milk
- 1 tsp honey (elective, for sweetness)

Directions:

1. Peel and pit the avocado.
2. Put your avocado, banana, almond milk, and honey (if wanted) inside a mixer.
3. Blend till smooth.

Per serving: Calories: 230kcal; Fat: 10 g; Carbs: 35 g; Protein: 3 g; Sodium: 100mg

112. *Watermelon and Cucumber Cooler*

Preparation time: 10 mins

Cooking time: 0 mins

Servings: 2

Ingredients:

- 2 teacups cubed watermelon
- 1/2 cucumber, skinned and cubed
- 1 tbsp fresh lime juice
- Fresh mint leaves for garnish

Directions:

1. Put your watermelon, cucumber, and lime juice inside a mixer.
2. Blend till smooth.
3. Spoon into glasses and top with a sprig of fresh mint.

Per serving: Calories: 50kcal; Fat: 0 g; Carbs: 12 g; Protein: 1 g; Sodium: 0mg

113. *Kiwi and Spinach Smoothie*

Preparation time: 5 mins
Cooking time: 0 mins
Servings: 1
Ingredients:

- 2 ripe kiwis, skinned and carved
- 1 teacup fresh spinach leaves
- 1/2 teacup unsweetened coconut water
- 1 tsp honey (elective, for sweetness)

Directions:

1. Put your kiwis, spinach, coconut water, and honey (if wanted) inside a mixer.
2. Blend till smooth.

Per serving: Calories: 130kcal; Fat: 1 g; Carbs: 33 g; Protein: 2 g; Sodium: 100mg

114. *Homemade Vegetable Juice*

Preparation time: 10 mins
Cooking time: 0 mins
Servings: 2
Ingredients:

- 2 large tomatoes
- 1 cucumber
- 2 stalks celery
- 1/2 lemon, juiced
- Tweak of black pepper

Directions:

1. Wash and chop the tomatoes, cucumber, and celery.
2. Run the vegetables through a juicer.
3. Place lemon juice and a tweak of black pepper for flavor.

Per serving: Calories: 40kcal; Fat: 0 g; Carbs: 10 g; Protein: 2 g; Sodium: 40mg

115. *Papaya and Coconut Water Smoothie*

Preparation time: 5 mins

Cooking time: 0 mins

Servings: 1

Ingredients:

- 1 teacup ripe papaya, cubed
- 1/2 teacup unsweetened coconut water
- 1/4 tsp fresh lime juice

Directions:

1. Put your papaya, coconut water, and lime juice inside a mixer.
2. Blend till smooth.

Per serving: Calories: 90kcal; Fat: 0 g; Carbs: 23 g; Protein: 1 g; Sodium: 100mg

116. *Blueberry and Almond Milk Smoothie*

Preparation time: 5 mins

Cooking time: 0 mins

Servings: 1

Ingredients:

- 1/2 teacup blueberries (fresh or frozen)
- 1/2 banana
- 1 teacup unsweetened almond milk
- 1 tbsp almond butter (elective, for creaminess)

Directions:

1. Place blueberries, banana, almond milk, and almond butter (if using) inside a mixer.
2. Blend till smooth.

Per serving: Calories: 140kcal; Fat: 6 g; Carbs: 22 g; Protein: 2 g; Sodium: 100mg

117. *Minty Fresh Lemonade*

Preparation time: 10 mins

Cooking time: 0 mins

Servings: 2

Ingredients:

- Juice of 2 lemons
- 2 teacups water
- Fresh mint leaves
- 1-2 tsps honey (elective, for sweetness)

Directions:

1. Inside a pitcher, blend lemon juice and water.
2. Include fresh mint leaves and honey (if wanted) for flavor.

3. Stir well and present over ice.

Per serving: Calories: 10kcal; Fat: 0 g; Carbs: 3 g; Protein: 0 g; Sodium: 0mg

118. *Green Detox Smoothie*

Preparation time: 5 mins

Cooking time: 0 mins

Servings: 1

Ingredients:

- 1 teacup fresh spinach leaves
- 1/2 cucumber, skinned and carved
- 1/2 green apple, carved
- 1/2 lemon, juiced
- 1/2 teacup unsweetened coconut water

Directions:

1. Place spinach, cucumber, green apple, lemon juice, and coconut water inside a mixer.
2. Blend till smooth.

Per serving: Calories: 70kcal; Fat: 0 g; Carbs: 17 g; Protein: 1 g; Sodium: 90mg

119. *Beet and Spinach Juice*

Preparation time: 10 mins

Cooking time: 0 mins

Servings: 2

Ingredients:

- 2 medium beets, skinned and severed
- 2 teacups fresh spinach leaves
- 1/2 lemon, juiced

Directions:

1. Run the beets and spinach through a juicer.
2. Include lemon juice for flavor.

Per serving: Calories: 70kcal; Fat: 0 g; Carbs: 17 g; Protein: 2 g; Sodium: 170mg

120. *Pineapple and Coconut Milk Smoothie*

Preparation time: 5 mins

Cooking time: 0 mins

Servings: 1

Ingredients:

- 1 teacup cubed pineapple
- 1/2 teacup unsweetened coconut milk
- 1/2 banana

Directions:

1. Place pineapple, coconut milk, and banana inside a mixer.
2. Blend till smooth.

Per serving: Calories: 200kcal; Fat: 8 g; Carbs: 36 g; Protein: 2 g; Sodium: 15mg

Special Considerations and Customizations

In this chapter, we'll explore how to adapt the DASH Diet to various situations and lifestyles. Whether you're looking to shed pounds, maintain an active lifestyle, or address specific age-related nutritional needs, the DASH Diet can be tailored to your unique circumstances. Additionally, we'll delve into how vegetarians and vegans can embrace DASH principles while managing sodium intake effectively.

Adapting DASH for Weight Loss: Tips and Strategies

The DASH Diet is not only effective for managing blood pressure and promoting heart health but can also be a valuable tool for weight loss. Here's how to tailor it for your weight loss goals:

1. **Caloric Intake:** Based on your age, gender, exercise level, and weight reduction objectives, calculate how many calories you need to consume each day to lose weight. Aim for a calorie deficit by taking in less energy than your body uses.

2. **Portion Control:** Exercise caution with portion sizes to avoid overindulging. Utilize smaller plates and containers as a visual aid to manage your portions effectively.

3. **Choose Low-Calorie DASH Foods:** Prioritize foods that are low in calories but still align with DASH principles, such as fruits, vegetables, lean proteins, and whole grains.

4. **Limit High-Calorie Foods:** While the DASH Diet encourages nutrient-dense foods, be mindful of high-calorie items like nuts and avocados. Consume them in moderation.

5. **Monitor Your Intake:** To track your daily food consumption and measure your improvement, keep a food journal. You can use this to determine your areas of improvement.

6. **Remain Hydrated:** Occasionally, hunger might be confused with thirst. Stay well-hydrated by consuming ample water throughout the day, which can help prevent unnecessary snacking.

7. **Frequent Physical Activity:** To improve general health and weight loss outcomes, combine the DASH Diet with regular exercise.

8. **Speak with a Dietitian:** For individualized advice and meal planning, think about scheduling a consultation with a registered dietitian who specializes in weight management.

DASH for Athletes: Fueling Your Active Lifestyle

Certain food requirements apply to athletes in order to support their performance and training. Here's how to customize the DASH Diet for active individuals:

1. **Increase Caloric Intake:** Athletes require more calories to fuel their workouts and recover. Determine your calorie requirements by considering your activity level and objectives.

2. **Carbohydrates for Energy:** Give precedence to complex carbohydrates like fruits, whole grains, and vegetables to supply long-lasting energy for your workouts.

3. **Protein for Muscle Repair:** To promote muscle growth and repair, include lean protein sources including fish, poultry, lean meats, and plant-based foods like beans and tofu.

4. **Hydration:** Drink plenty of water before, during, and after physical activity. For longer workouts, consider a sports drink to restore electrolytes in addition to drinking plenty of water.

5. **Snack Smart:** Incorporate healthy snacks like fruit, yogurt, or a handful of nuts to refuel between meals and maintain energy levels.

6. **Post-Workout Nutrition:** After intense workouts, consume a balanced meal rich in carbohydrates and protein to aid recovery.

7. **Supplements:** If needed, discuss the use of supplements like protein powder or electrolyte tablets with a healthcare provider or sports nutritionist.

8. **Take Note of Your Body:** Observe your body's signals of hunger and fullness, and modify your food intake accordingly. Every athlete's needs are unique.

9. **Periodization:** Adjust your nutrition plan based on your training cycle. For example, increase carbohydrates leading up to a race or event for peak performance.

10. **Consult a Sports Dietitian:** For personalized guidance, consider consulting a sports dietitian who can create a tailored nutrition plan to meet your athletic goals.

DASH for Seniors: Nutritional Needs as You Age

Our dietary requirements vary with age, therefore it's critical to maintain a healthy diet for overall well-++being. The DASH Diet can be particularly beneficial for seniors, as it focuses on heart health and blood pressure management, which are key concerns as we grow older.

As seniors age, their nutritional requirements evolve. Here are some essential nutritional needs and considerations for seniors:

1. **Caloric Intake:** Metabolism tends to slow down with age, meaning fewer calories are needed. However, the need for essential nutrients remains high, so it's crucial to form every calorie count by choosing nutrient-dense foods.

2. **Protein:** Maintaining muscle mass becomes more challenging as we age. To maintain muscle health and avoid sarcopenia (muscle loss), an adequate protein diet is essential.

3. **Fiber:** Digestive issues become more common with age. A diet abundant in fiber sourced from vegetables, fruits, & whole grains can be beneficial in preventing constipation and promoting digestive health.

4. **Calcium and Vitamin D:** Bone health is a significant concern for seniors, as the risk of osteoporosis increases. Calcium & vitamin D are essential for maintaining strong bones.

5. **B Vitamins:** These vitamins, particularly B12, can become less efficiently absorbed by the body as we age. Energy production and nerve function depend on vitamin B12.

6. **Hydration:** Due to their diminished sense of thirst, seniors are more likely to become dehydrated. Maintaining proper hydration is fundamental for overall well-being and can play a role in preventing urinary tract infections and alleviating constipation.

7. **Sodium Reduction:** Hypertension (high blood pressure) is more prevalent among older adults. Reducing sodium intake is crucial for controlling blood pressure and lowering the risk of heart disease.

Adapting the DASH Diet for Seniors

Here's how seniors can adapt the DASH Diet to meet their specific nutritional needs:

1. **Seek Guidance from a Healthcare Provider:** Prior to implementing substantial dietary modifications, it is crucial to seek guidance from a healthcare provider or registered dietitian. They can evaluate your specific health situation and offer tailored recommendations.

2. **Caloric Adjustment:** In general, older persons require less calories than younger ones. Adjust portion sizes to meet your caloric needs while maintaining nutrient density.

3. **Protein-Rich Foods:** Include foods high in protein in your diet, such as fish, poultry, beans, lean meats, and low-fat dairy. These help preserve muscle mass and support overall health.

4. **Fruits and Vegetables:** To ensure you are getting enough vitamins, minerals, and fiber in your diet, keep putting an emphasis on fruits and vegetables. Try to find a range of vibrant options.

5. **Whole Grains:** Choose whole grains to sustain stable energy levels and promote intestinal health, such as brown rice, whole wheat bread, and oats.

6. **Dairy or Dairy Alternatives:** Ensure you get enough calcium and vitamin D for bone health. Choose low-fat or fat-free dairy products or fortified dairy alternatives like almond or soy milk.

7. **Fluid Intake:** Stay vigilant about staying hydrated. Develop the practice of drinking water throughout the day and eat foods high in hydration, such as fruits, vegetables, and soups.

8. **Sodium Awareness:** Consider your sodium intake and select options with reduced or no added salt when possible. Use herbs & spices to flavor foods instead of salt.

9. **Regular Physical Activity:** Integrate a well-rounded diet with consistent physical activity to sustain muscle strength, flexibility, and overall mobility.

10. **Medication Interactions:** It's critical to understand that various drugs may interact with particular foods. To safeguard your health, have a conversation with your healthcare provider about your medication regimen to ensure that your diet doesn't hinder the effectiveness of your medications.

11. **Regular Check-Ups:** Make sure to arrange periodic check-ups with your healthcare provider to keep track of your overall health, which includes monitoring blood pressure, cholesterol levels, and nutritional status.

Vegetarian and Vegan DASH: Plant-Based Alternatives

Adopting a vegetarian or vegan lifestyle while following the DASH Diet is entirely possible and can offer numerous health benefits. Whether you choose to avoid animal products for ethical, environmental, or health reasons, you can still relish the advantages of the DASH Diet. Here's how to create a plant-based DASH plan:

Plant-Based Protein Sources:

- **Legumes:** Beans, lentils, & chickpeas are excellent sources of protein and fiber. They are adaptable and go well with salads, stews, and soups
- **Tofu and Tempeh:** Soy-based products are abundant in protein and versatile, suitable for a range of dishes such as stir-fries and sandwiches.
- **Nuts and Seeds:** For healthy fats and protein, include unsalted nuts and seeds in your diet, such as flaxseeds, chia seeds, walnuts, and almonds.
- **Seitan:** Seitan, sometimes referred to as wheat meat or wheat gluten, is a high-protein meat alternative that works well in a variety of cuisines.

Whole Grains:

- **Quinoa:** This grain is high in fiber and a full source of protein. It can serve as a side dish or as the foundation for grain containers.
- **Brown Rice:** For more fiber and minerals, choose brown rice instead of white rice.
- **Whole Wheat:** Opt for whole wheat pasta, bread, and other products to increase your intake of whole grains.

Fruits and Vegetables:

- **Leafy Greens:** Kale, spinach, Swiss chard, and collard greens are nutrient-dense and can be used in salads, smoothies, or sautéed dishes.
- **Berries:** Rich in antioxidants, blackberries, raspberries, and blueberries are delectable additions to breakfast or snacks.
- **Colorful Vegetables:** To guarantee a varied vitamin intake, incorporate a range of vibrant veggies into your meals, such as tomatoes, bell peppers, and carrots.

Dairy Alternatives:

- **Plant-Based Milks:** For calcium and vitamin D, go for unsweetened almond milk, oat milk, soy milk, or other plant-based milk substitutes.
- **Vegan Cheese:** Dairy cheese can be substituted with a variety of vegan cheese options that are manufactured from almonds or soy.

Fats:

- **Healthy Oils:** Use heart-healthy oils like olive oil, canola oil, and avocado oil in your cooking and for salad dressings.
- **Avocado:** Avocado provides a rich source of healthy fats and can be utilized in sandwiches, salads, or as a flavorful topping.

Managing Sodium: Techniques for Salt Reduction

Reducing sodium intake is a central aspect of the DASH Diet, as excessive sodium can contribute to high blood pressure. Here are some techniques for effectively managing sodium:

1. **Read Food Labels:** Observe the amount of salt listed on food labels. Seek for goods with the labels "no-salt-added" or "low-sodium."

2. **Use Herbs and Spices:** Flavour your food with herbs, spices, and other flavorful seasonings like garlic, onion, lemon juice, and vinegar instead of salt.

3. **Cook at Home:** You can regulate how much salt is in your food when you cook it yourself. Use less salt when cooking, and try salt-free seasoning blends.

4. **Rinse Canned Foods:** To lower the sodium level in canned beans, vegetables, or other products, give them a thorough rinse under running water.

5. **Reduce Your Consumption of Processed Foods:** Convenience and processed foods frequently have high salt content. Reduce how much of these things you use.

6. **Select Low-Sodium Products:** Whenever possible, choose low-sodium sauces, broths, and condiments.

7. **Gradual Reduction:** To help your taste buds adjust to lower sodium levels, gradually cut back on your salt intake.

8. **Be Mindful When Eating Out:** Request that foods be made with less salt when dining at restaurants, and refrain from adding additional salt at the table.

9. **Fresh and Frozen Foods:** Prioritize fresh or frozen fruits and vegetables over canned options, as they tend to have lower sodium levels.

10. **Keep a Sodium Diary:** Keep track of your daily sodium intake to ensure you're meeting your sodium reduction goals.

Beyond the Plate

This chapter explores the vital impact that physical activity and exercise play when paired with a healthy diet—more particularly, the DASH Diet. While nutrition is a cornerstone of health, a well-rounded approach includes regular physical activity to maximize the benefits for heart health, blood pressure control, and overall well-being.

Exercise and Physical Activity: Complementing the DASH Diet

The DASH Diet is well known for its ability to lower high blood pressure and improve heart health mostly by altering one's diet. However, to achieve the best results and maintain overall health, it's essential to pair the DASH Diet with a regular exercise regimen. Here's why exercise is vital and how to incorporate it effectively:

1. **Synergy of Diet and Exercise**

Combining a heart-healthy diet with physical activity creates a powerful synergy. Exercise can enhance the benefits of the DASH Diet by further reducing blood pressure, promoting weight management, and improving cardiovascular health.

2. **Blood Pressure Control**

Exercises that focus on strength and aerobics have been demonstrated to help decrease blood pressure. Regular physical activity can complement the DASH Diet's impact on hypertension.

3. **Weight Management**

Sustaining a healthy weight is vital for heart health. Exercise plays a significant role by burning calories and promoting the development of lean muscle, which simplifies the attainment and maintenance of a healthy weight.

4. **Cardiovascular Health**

Exercise improves cardiovascular fitness by enhancing heart and lung function. It can lower the chance of stroke, heart disease, and other cardiovascular disorders.

5. **Blood Sugar Regulation**

Being physically active lowers the risk of type 2 diabetes, which is directly related to heart health via regulating blood sugar levels.

6. **Stress Reduction**

Exercise has stress-reducing effects, which can indirectly benefit heart health by lowering stress-related hormones and promoting relaxation.

7. **Improved Mood and Mental Health**

Consistent physical activity triggers the release of endorphins, which have the potential to enhance mood and alleviate symptoms of depression and anxiety, ultimately contributing to overall well-being.

8. **Enhanced Quality of Life**

Exercise increases mobility, flexibility, and strength, allowing for a better quality of life as we age.

9. **Types of Exercise**

- **Aerobic Exercise:** Walking, jogging, cycling, swimming, and dancing are exercises that increase endurance and cardiovascular fitness. Aim for almost 150 mins of moderate-intensity aerobic exercise or 75 mins of vigorous-intensity aerobic exercise each week.
- **Strength Training:** To promote muscle growth and maintenance, incorporate resistance training into your program by using weights, resistance bands, or bodyweight movements. Incorporate strength training activities for the main muscle groups about twice a week.
- **Flexibility and Balance:** Yoga, tai chi, and stretching routines improve flexibility and balance, reducing the risk of falls and injuries, especially important for older adults.

10. Combining Diet and Exercise

Pairing the DASH Diet with regular exercise optimizes heart health. A well-rounded diet furnishes essential nutrients, while regular physical activity enhances heart health and boosts circulation.

11. Getting Started

If you're new to exercise or haven't been active for a while, start slowly and gradually increase intensity and duration. Before starting a new fitness regimen, especially if you have any health issues already, you should consult a healthcare professional.

12. Make It Enjoyable

Select activities that you find enjoyable to ensure that exercise becomes a lasting and consistent part of your daily routine. Find something you enjoy doing, whether it's dancing, gardening, hiking, or team sports.

13. Consistency Matters

Consistency is key. Aim for regular, ongoing physical activity to reap the long-term health benefits. Make a timetable that suits your needs and follow it.

14. Listen to Your Body

Observe the cues your body sends you. If you encounter pain, discomfort, or unusual symptoms while exercising, it's crucial to halt and seek guidance from a healthcare professional.

15. Accountability and Support

Think about working out with a friend or becoming a part of a fitness group to enhance motivation and ensure accountability in your exercise routine.

16. Monitor Progress

Monitor your fitness development and acknowledge your accomplishments as you go. Keeping track of your accomplishments helps increase drive.

Along with following the DASH Diet, regular exercise can greatly improve your heart health and general well-being. Together, these two pillars offer a thorough plan for living an active and healthy life. Remember that every step counts, and it's never too late to start reaping the benefits of a balanced diet and physical activity.

30 Day Meal Plan

Day	Breakfast	Lunch	Dinner	Dessert
1	Banana and Spinach Smoothie	Tuna Salad with Mixed Greens	Grilled Tofu with Peanut Sauce	Mixed Berries with A Sprinkle of Cinnamon
2	Veggie Frittata with Herbs	Turkey and Vegetable Stir-Fry	Baked Cod with Mediterranean Herbs	Sliced Apple with Almond Butter
3	Blueberry and Spinach Smoothie Bowl	Quinoa and Spinach Stuffed Peppers	Mushroom and Spinach Stuffed Portobello Mushrooms	Baked Sweet Potato Fries
4	Sweet Potato Hash with Avocado	Chickpea and Spinach Curry	Spaghetti Aglio E Olio with Spinach	Chia Seed Pudding with Berries
5	Mediterranean Breakfast Bowl	Spinach and Feta Stuffed Chicken Breast	Baked Salmon with Lemon and Dill	Dark Chocolate Covered Almonds
6	Overnight Chia Seed Pudding with Berries	Quinoa and Black Bean Stuffed Acorn Squash	Lemon Garlic Chicken with Asparagus	Greek Yogurt Bark with Fruit
7	Apple Cinnamon Oatmeal	Greek Salad with Grilled Chicken	Grilled Chicken with Spinach and Tomato Salsa	Banana Slices with Peanut Butter
8	Almond Flour Banana Muffins	Caprese Sandwich With Pesto	Quinoa-Stuffed Bell Peppers	Sliced Cucumber with Olive Oil and Vinegar
9	Vegetable Omelet with A Side of Oranges	Mediterranean Quinoa Salad	Honey Mustard Glazed Salmon	Air-Popped Popcorn with Herbs
10	Egg White and Veggie Scramble	Mixed Bean Salad with Herbs	Spinach and Mushroom Risotto	Roasted Chickpeas with Herbs
11	Berry and Spinach Breakfast Salad	Turkey and Avocado Wrap	Lentil and Spinach Curry	Banana Slices with Peanut Butter
12	Avocado Toast with Tomato and Herbs	Quinoa and Spinach Stuffed Peppers	Grilled Turkey Burger with Avocado	Whole Wheat Banana Bread
13	Scrambled Eggs with Spinach and Feta	Chickpea and Spinach Curry	Baked Zucchini Boats with Ground Turkey	Greek Yogurt Bark with Fruit
14	Quinoa Porridge with Almond Butter	Tuna Salad with Mixed Greens	Spaghetti Squash with Tomato and	Almond and Date Energy Bites

			Basil Sauce	
15	Whole Wheat Pancakes with Fresh Fruit	Hummus and Veggie Wrap	Vegetable Stir-Fry with Brown Rice	Berry Smoothie with Spinach
16	Breakfast Quinoa with Pecans and Raisins	Spinach and Feta Stuffed Chicken Breast	Mediterranean Couscous Salad	Sliced Cucumber with Olive Oil and Vinegar
17	Cottage Cheese with Pineapple and Walnuts	Mediterranean Quinoa Salad	Grilled Chicken with Spinach and Tomato Salsa	Baked Sweet Potato Fries
18	Mediterranean Breakfast Bowl	Quinoa and Spinach Stuffed Peppers	Mushroom and Spinach Stuffed Portobello Mushrooms	Chia Seed Pudding with Berries
19	Banana and Spinach Smoothie	Caprese Sandwich With Pesto	Quinoa-Stuffed Bell Peppers	Dark Chocolate Covered Almonds
20	Blueberry and Spinach Smoothie Bowl	Turkey and Avocado Wrap	Baked Cod with Mediterranean Herbs	Greek Yogurt Bark with Fruit
21	Sweet Potato Hash with Avocado	Mixed Bean Salad with Herbs	Spaghetti Aglio E Olio with Spinach	Sliced Apple with Almond Butter
22	Overnight Chia Seed Pudding with Berries	Greek Salad with Grilled Chicken	Lemon Garlic Chicken with Asparagus	Mixed Berries with A Sprinkle of Cinnamon
23	Apple Cinnamon Oatmeal	Tuna Salad with Mixed Greens	Grilled Turkey Burger with Avocado	Banana Slices with Peanut Butter
24	Almond Flour Banana Muffins	Quinoa and Spinach Stuffed Peppers	Lentil and Spinach Curry	Baked Sweet Potato Fries
25	Vegetable Omelet with A Side of Oranges	Chickpea and Spinach Curry	Baked Zucchini Boats with Ground Turkey	Chia Seed Pudding with Berries
26	Egg White and Veggie Scramble	Caprese Sandwich With Pesto	Mushroom and Spinach Stuffed Portobello Mushrooms	Dark Chocolate Covered Almonds
27	Berry and Spinach Breakfast Salad	Greek Salad with Grilled Chicken	Spaghetti Squash with Tomato and Basil Sauce	Greek Yogurt Bark with Fruit
28	Avocado Toast with Tomato and Herbs	Turkey and Avocado Wrap	Honey Mustard Glazed Salmon	Sliced Apple with Almond Butter

29	Scrambled Eggs with Spinach and Feta	Quinoa and Spinach Stuffed Peppers	Vegetable Stir-Fry with Brown Rice	Mixed Berries with A Sprinkle of Cinnamon
30	Quinoa Porridge with Almond Butter	Mixed Bean Salad with Herbs	Grilled Chicken with Spinach and Tomato Salsa	Chia Seed Pudding with Berries

Conversion Table

Volume Equivalents (Liquid)

US Standard	US Standard (oz.)	Metric (approximate)
2 tbsps	1 fl. oz.	30 milliliter
¼ teacup	2 fl. oz.	60 milliliter
½ teacup	4 fl. oz.	120 milliliter
1 teacup	8 fl. oz.	240 milliliter
1½ teacups	12 fl. oz.	355 milliliter
2 teacups or 1 pint	16 fl. oz.	475 milliliter
4 teacups or 1 quart	32 fl. oz.	1 Liter
1 gallon	128 fl. oz.	4 Liter

Volume Equivalents (Dry)

US Standard	Metric (approximate)
⅛ tsp	0.5 milliliter
¼ tsp	1 milliliter
½ tsp	2 milliliter
¾ tsp	4 milliliter
1 tsp	5 milliliter
1 tbsp	15 milliliter
¼ teacup	59 milliliter
⅓ teacup	79 milliliter
½ teacup	118 milliliter
⅔ teacup	156 milliliter
¾ teacup	177 milliliter
1 teacup	235 milliliter
2 teacups or 1 pint	475 milliliter
3 teacups	700 milliliter
4 teacups or 1 quart	1 Liter

Oven Temperatures

Fahrenheit (F)	Celsius (C) (approximate)
250 deg.F	120 deg.C
300 deg.F	150 deg.C
325 deg.F	165 deg.C
350 deg.F	180 deg.C

375 deg.F	190 deg.C
400 deg.F	200 deg.C
425 deg.F	220 deg.C
450 deg.F	230 deg.C

Weight Equivalents

US Standard	Metric (approximate)
1 tbsp	15 gm
½ oz.	15 gm
1 oz.	30 gm
2 oz.	60 gm
4 oz.	115 gm
8 oz.	225 gm
12 oz.	340 gm
16 oz. or 1 lb.	455 gm

Conclusion

In conclusion, the DASH diet has proven itself as a valuable and real dietary tactic for promoting better health and well-being. Its emphasis on whole, nutrient-rich foods, and its ability to reduce the risk of heart disease, hypertension, and other chronic conditions make it a standout choice for those seeking a sustainable and balanced way of eating.

The DASH diet is not just about restricting certain foods; it's about making mindful and informed choices that benefit your overall health. Combining these two pillars yields a comprehensive plan for living an active and healthy life.

For those looking to adopt the DASH diet and explore its culinary possibilities, I encourage you to dive into the recipes featured in the book. These recipes have been carefully crafted to align with the principles of the DASH diet while ensuring that flavor and enjoyment are not compromised. There is something for every appetite, from savory main courses to decadent desserts, and from light salads to filling soups.

Thus, don't be afraid to attempt these dishes and start your journey to a healthy you. By adopting the DASH diet as part of your lifestyle, you can make substantial strides in lowering your risk of chronic diseases, enhancing your blood pressure, and attaining improved overall well-being.

Lastly, I would want to sincerely thank all of the readers for joining us on this adventure. Your commitment to improving your health and making informed dietary choices is commendable. I hope that this book has provided you with valuable insights and practical tools to support your DASH diet journey.

Always remember that your health is an priceless asset, and proactively caring for it is a remarkable gift to both yourself and your loved ones.

Thank you for your trust and dedication. Here's to a healthier, happier, and more vibrant you. Happy cooking and happy, healthy eating!

Index

Made in the USA
Coppell, TX
08 February 2024